Praise for *Sustainable Medicine*

"Dr. Sarah Myhill's honest voice is a beacon of light and hope in a world where conventional medicine is the third leading cause of death in the United States, surpassed only by cancer and cardiovascular disease. She simplifies disease as a lack of raw materials, blocked/damaged powerhouses, and membrane issues (shape and flexibility as well as permeability). Dr. Myhill empowers the patient by offering a thoughtful road map, inspired by her brilliant analogies, to restore proper mitochondrial function that ultimately leads to health and vitality."

—DR. NASHA WINTERS,
coauthor of *The Metabolic Approach to Cancer*

"Rather than helping people achieve health by getting to the root cause of disease, profit-driven conventional medicine perpetuates disease by treating symptoms with an endless panoply of pharmaceutical medications. A trip to the doctor will often make you sicker, not healthier. While many people understand this on some level, it can be hard to know where to go from there. That's why Dr. Sarah Myhill's *Sustainable Medicine* is so valuable. She not only critiques twenty-first century medical practice for its misplaced priorities, but she offers readers a far more valuable alternative: the tools to understand their symptoms and the mechanisms at play that give rise to them, so that 'health care consumers' can instead be empowered agents of their own well-being."

—TOM COWAN, MD,
author of *Human Heart, Cosmic Heart*

"Dr. Sarah Myhill provides us with not only a critique of current medical practice but also a detailed viable alternative, which she aptly refers to as 'sustainable medicine'—sustainable because the focus is on the underlying causes of disease rather than merely the management of symptoms. The approach is highly integrative. Dr. Myhill utilizes nutritional medicine, lifestyle interventions, appropriate clinical tests, and, yes, were necessary, conventional medical treatments. *Sustainable Medicine* is a manual for good health in the twenty-first century. It makes a great deal of sense, starting from the basis of what constitutes good health and working up to many more detailed areas. Dr. Myhill also dispels a number of medical myths along the way—what we are told about cholesterol, low-fat diets, problems with digestion—and describes the real causes of various conditions prevalent today. The detailed advice about nutritional supplementation with appropriate dosages throughout the book is also particularly beneficial.

"Despite the immense contribution Dr. Myhill has given to the advancement of medical practice, she remains incredibly humble, clearly valuing the insights provided by patients and continuing to learn and make appropriate modifications to various protocols."

—JUSTIN SMITH, author of *Statin Nation*; producer of the documentary films *Statin Nation* and *Statin Nation II*

"This book grabbed my attention from the first page and kept me fascinated right to the very end. Dr. Myhill sees many of the current 'diagnostic' and 'treatment' practices in modern medicine to be unsustainable because they do not actually deal with the real underlying causes of ill health. This argument is explained so clearly and carefully that it is impossible to disagree with it. God! I hope the medical profession sit up and listen.

"Dr. Myhill at one point describes this book as '. . . the end result of 30 years of trial and error'. This description doesn't come close to the achievement that it represents. She has managed to pull off the near impossible and has packaged up an overall blueprint for good health. This blueprint can help patients recover from a wide range of conditions and forms a platform for future good health. It's a *tour de force*!

"If you are sick of being sick then this book could transform your life. However, it can also be used by people who are fit and well in order to remain so to a ripe old age."

—PAUL ROBINSON, author of *Recovering with T3*

"Dr. Myhill addresses the principle causes for the current epidemic of chronic diseases in the Western World and outlines in her unique, no-nonsense way how to explain, prevent, diagnose and successfully treat those conditions for which conventional medicine currently only has an ever increasing amount of potentially dangerous medicines to offer.

"This book is an invitation for patients and practitioners alike to move away from a culture of ignorance, restrictive guidelines and blame and to make informed decisions and take responsibility for their own health again."

—DR. FRANZISKA MEUSCHEL, MD, PhD, ND, LFhom

"This is Sarah's Principia; the science, the medicine and the under-standing are all hers. My contributions as editor were limited to the typographical, the organisational, and some of the quotations. It was a pleasure to be involved in this project both to witness how a truly unique, caring and great mind comes to an understanding of the labyrinth of modern dis-ease processes and then also to be party to the thought patterns that the said mind undertakes in order to develop sustainable treatments for those diseases. It is not for the editor to advise the reader, but I shall break with protocol; perhaps it is personal to me, but I gained most from this book by reading it in one sitting and would suggest that, if possible, others do likewise. Thereafter one can 'dip in' at will. Your Good Health!"

—CRAIG ROBINSON, MA (Oxon) ACA

Sustainable Medicine

Whistle-Blowing on 21st-Century Medical Practice

Dr. Sarah Myhill, MB, BS

Chelsea Green Publishing
White River Junction, Vermont

Original edition published in 2015 by Hammersmith Books, London, United Kingdom,
under exclusive license for all formats, languages and territories.

This edition published by Chelsea Green Publishing, 2018. This edition is authorized for sale
only in North America.

Disclaimer: The information contained in this book is for educational purposes only. It is the result of
the study and the experience of the author. Whilst the information and advice offered are believed to be
true and accurate at the time of going to press, neither the author nor the publisher can accept any legal
responsibility or liability for any errors or omissions that may have been made or for any adverse effects
which may occur as a result of following the recommendations given herein. Always consult a qualified
medical practitioner if you have any concerns regarding your health.

Editor: Craig Robinson

Printed in the United States of America.
First printing February, 2018.
10 9 8 7 6 5 4 3 2 1   18 19 20 21 22

Our Commitment to Green Publishing
Chelsea Green sees publishing as a tool for cultural change and ecological stewardship. We strive to align our
book manufacturing practices with our editorial mission and to reduce the impact of our business enterprise
in the environment. We print our books and catalogs on chlorine-free recycled paper, using vegetable-based
inks whenever possible. This book may cost slightly more because it was printed on paper that contains
recycled fiber, and we hope you'll agree that it's worth it. Chelsea Green is a member of the Green Press
Initiative (www.greenpressinitiative.org), a nonprofit coalition of publishers, manufacturers, and authors
working to protect the world's endangered forests and conserve natural resources. *Sustainable Medicine* was
printed on paper supplied by Thomson-Shore that contains 100% postconsumer recycled fiber.

Library of Congress Cataloging-in-Publication Data
Names: Myhill, Sarah, author.
Title: Sustainable medicine : whistle-blowing on 21st-century medical practice / Dr. Sarah Myhill, MB, BS.
Description: White River Junction, Vermont : Chelsea Green Publishing, 2018. | Originally published in
  2015 by Hammersmith Books, London, United Kingdom. | Includes bibliographical references and index.
Identifiers: LCCN 2017051100 | ISBN 9781603587891 (pbk.) | ISBN 9781603587907 (ebook)
Subjects: LCSH: Medicine—Philosophy. | BISAC: MEDICAL / Holistic Medicine. | MEDICAL /
  Nutrition. | MEDICAL / Health Care Delivery. | HEALTH & FITNESS / Holism. | HEALTH &
  FITNESS / General.
Classification: LCC R723 .M94 2018 | DDC 610.1--dc23
LC record available at https://lccn.loc.gov/2017051100

Chelsea Green Publishing
85 North Main Street, Suite 120
White River Junction, VT 05001
(802) 295-6300
www.chelseagreen.com

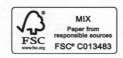

*This book is dedicated to my lovely patients
who embraced my practice of medicine and stuck
with me even when my ideas were rotten ones.
Bless them all!
I am so sorry that it took me so long
to start to identify the paths to recovery.*

Contents

Acknowledgements

If I have seen further it is by standing on the shoulders of giants.

SIR ISAAC NEWTON (1642–1727)

The intellectual giants who guided me through the early days, and to whom I am forever grateful, include Dr Len McEwen (who developed EPD – see page 199) and the four authors of *Environmental Medicine in Clinical Practice*, namely Dr Honor Anthony, Dr Sybil Birtwistle, Dr Keith Eaton and Dr Jonathan Maberley. Meanwhile, I have never spent time with Dr Patrick Kingsley, Dr John Mansfield or Dr David Freed and failed to come away with a new idea or a solution to a clinical problem.

Dr Ellen Grant put me right early on over the dangers of the Pill and HRT. I spent hours talking to Dr Dick van Steenis and learned so much about pollution of the environment and its medical consequences. I believe that between them these two doctors, in recent history, have done more for the Health of the Nation than any others.

The giant amongst the giants is Dr John McLaren-Howard, from whom I have learned more than from all others put together. I can ask the difficult questions but it takes a genius to come up with answers which are clinically applicable, relevant and available. His knowledge is encyclopaedic and he is so generous with his time and energy.

Dr Norman Booth had sufficient faith to collate hundreds of statistics and apply the necessary academic rigor to turn those into publishable material to demonstrate the power of nutritional medicine. Thank you, Norman!

I judge the worth of a lecture or a book by the degree to which it shapes my thinking and changes my clinical practice. New ideas which have been original, instructive and helpful have come from:

Professor Guy Abraham (iodine)
Nina Barnes (Foresight work – preconceptual care)
Dr Eleonore Blaurock-Busch (chelation therapy and heavy metal toxicity)
Dr Thomas Borody (gut flora and faecal bacteriotherapy)

Professor Jonathan Brostoff (allergy and immunology)
Dr Sam Brown (intravenous magnesium therapy)
Dr Natasha Campbell-McBride (probiotics and GAPS diet)
Rachael Carson (*Silent Spring* – organochlorines)
Dr Stepen Davies (nutritional medicine)
Colonel Danny Goodwin Jones (trace elements)
Stephen Jay Gould (evolutionary biology)
Dr Abraham Hoffer (psychiatric disease)
Professor Malcolm Hooper (Gulf War syndrome)
Sir Albert Howard ('An Agricultural Testament' – organic farming)
Professor Vyvyan Howard (foetal pathology)
Rich van Konynenburg (methylation cycle)
Dr William Kaufman (arthritis)
Professor Nick Lane (evolutionary biology)
Professor Katsunari Nishihara (fermenting brain)
Dr Richard Mackarness (allergy and addiction)
Dr John Mansfield (allergy and nutrition)
Dr Michael Moseley (5:2 diet)
Rex Newnham (boron and arthritis)
Professor Martin Pall (pro-inflammatory NO/ON/OO cycle)
Mark Purdey (prion disorders and chemical poisoning)
Dr Uffe Ravnskov (cholesterol does not cause arterial disease)
Paul Robinson (T3 hypothyroidism)
Dr Yehuda Schoenfeld (autoimmune diseases)
Dr Gabriela Segura (ketogenic diet)
Dr Stephen Sinatra (mitochondrial dysfunction)
Dr Gordon Skinner (treatment of hypothyroidism)
Dr Reinhold Vieth (vitamin D)
Professor Lewis Wolpert (foetal development)
Dr Jonathan Wright (allergy and nutrition)
And many others

Medical practice is called that for good reason – the poor patients suffer whilst we doctors practise. A million thanks are due to my long-suffering patients who put up with, and stuck with, the difficult regimes that I imposed on them. It is the patients who do not respond to the bleedin' obvious who suffer most but from whom I have learnt most.

Finally, a major thank you to Terry Ellison, who built and maintained my website with his expertise given free and freely, and to my editor Craig

Robinson, first-class mathematician and logical brain, who helped me to turn my clinical meanderings into an understandable and coherent form. I would not have won my intellectual battles without his brilliant and logical mind.

Who am I?

I qualified as a doctor from the Middlesex Hospital Medical School in 1981 (Medicine with Honours). I went straight into NHS General Practice and worked there for 20 years. Since 2000 I have worked as a private GP. For 17 years I was the Honorary Secretary of the British Society for Ecological Medicine ('the Society', renamed from the British Society for Allergy, Environmental and Nutritional Medicine), a medical society interested in looking at causes of disease and treating through diet, vitamins and minerals, and through avoiding toxic stress.

My interest in the causes of disease and the underlying mechanisms of such started with chronic fatigue syndrome (CFS/ME). Together with Dr John McLaren-Howard of Acumen Laboratory and Dr Norman Booth of Mansfield College, Oxford, I co-authored three scientific papers studying the link between CFS/ME and mitochondrial dysfunction. These papers were published in the *International Journal of Clinical and Experimental Medicine* in 2009, 2012 and 2013[1] and are described more fully in my first book, *Diagnosing and Treating Chronic Fatigue Syndrome – it's mitochondria, not hypochondria.*

Although these papers concerned CFS, they were also, in a deeper sense, the crystallisation of my clinical experience, spanning decades of treating many other modern diseases. The combination of my academic ventures, along with the associated practical applications across the full range of these diseases, led me inexorably to some key conclusions.

The ideas on mitochondria contained within my CFS medical papers dovetail, in a biologically plausible way, with emerging ideas on immune activation and inflammation as causes of disease. What had become clear to me over the years was that the vast majority of modern disease could be explained in terms of the twin drivers of poor energy delivery mechanisms and inflammation. Both of these drivers of disease are a consequence of modern Western lifestyles, as characterised by nutritional deficiencies, toxic stress and infectious loads. So evolved this book, *Sustainable Medicine*, as a way of explaining the applications of the ideas, as expounded in my academic writings, to many other modern disease processes.

In reality, of course, I have been writing this book in my head for the entirety of my medical career. It is the summation and culmination of who I am and what I do. I am a naturally inquisitive person and, with the help of my patients and their intelligent questions and unfaltering desire for answers, I hope that the results of my curiosity contained in this book may help the many sufferers of modern diseases, far too many of whom currently languish on long-term 'symptom squashing' medications.

I have two daughters, Ruth and Claire, now grown up and working. My hobbies have all to do with daughters, horses, dogs and gardening. In the winter I hunt, in spring and autumn I go team chasing with occasional point-to-pointing. I run annual long-distance rides across and around Wales. These are for big kids, like me, and younger versions.

DR SARAH MYHILL
2015

It's all about asking the question 'why?'

I keep six honest serving men
(They taught me all I knew)
Their names are What and Why and When
And How and Where and Who.

RUDYARD KIPLING (1865–1936)

Lets start with the bleeding obvious – when all else fails, use your brain.

DR ADA MARION DANSIE, my grandmother and
Medical Consultant to George Bernard Shaw

Five years at medical school followed by one year in hospital jobs do little to prepare a doctor for the real world. I had no answers to the early questions thrown up by NHS General Practice – 'Why do I have high blood pressure?' 'Why do I get such awful headaches?' 'Why am I depressed?' Correct conventional answers to these questions are deficiency of, respectively, anti-hypertensive drugs, painkillers and SSRIs. But this is not the 'why' of the matter. Indeed, it is hardly even the 'what' of the matter. Masking the symptoms does not explain them. The clues, which the symptoms represent, have been missed and the investigative detective work, which should have resulted from those clues, has been left undone.

The world is full of obvious things which nobody by any chance ever observes.

Sherlock Holmes (*The Hound of the Baskervilles*
by Sir Arthur Conan Doyle)

One year on and I was breast-feeding my daughter Ruth. She had terrible three-month colic and all I could do to lessen the screams was to walk round the house, all night, with her in my arms. My husband Nick's reaction was, 'You're the effing doctor – you sort it out.' He was right. It was not until I stumbled across advice for me to give up all dairy products that the problem was resolved. So too was my chronic sinusitis and rhinitis. At the time this was a momentous and life-changing discovery – but this information was nowhere to be found in the medical textbooks.

Thirty years later, this common cause and effect is still nowhere to be found in the medical textbooks. I worried about not knowing causation. I had been trained to elicit clinical symptoms and signs and recognise clinical pictures, but actually what patients wanted to know was why. What did they need to do to put things right? My standard line had been, 'Well, let's do a blood test and come back next week.' This gave me time to rifle anxiously through my lecture notes and textbooks looking for answers. The answers my patients wanted were not there. It came as a great relief to me to find out that my patients really did not mind me telling them I did not know! Thankfully, they rated my ability to care higher than my ability to know all the answers. Thankfully, too, they were happy to help me with my researches and act as willing guinea pigs with the dietary and lifestyle experiments that actually addressed the root causes of their problems.

The investigation of a patient should be like a detective story – 90 per cent of the clues come from the history and 10 per cent from the examination. Tests may confirm or refute the hypothesis – because every diagnosis is just a hypothesis. Then, once the diagnosis has been further corroborated by test results, it has to be put to the ultimate test. The ultimate test is response to treatment. Is the patient better? If not, then the diagnosis is wrong.

Exitus acta probat. (The result validates the deeds.)

OVID (43 BC–17/18 AD)

The word 'doctor' originates from the Latin verb 'doce', meaning 'I teach'. My job is to teach my patients to heal themselves and supply them with the necessary tools to do so. The doctor should be the interface between the hard science and the idiosyncratic patient – the practice of medicine is an Art.

Doctors routinely confuse the making of diagnoses with what are merely the descriptions of symptoms and clinical pictures, neither of which constitute a true diagnosis. Examples include hypertension (aka high blood pressure), asthma, irritable bowel syndrome and arthritis, all of which terms are in fact descriptions of symptoms and none of which is an actual diagnosis of the underlying cause. Clinical pictures include Parkinson's disease, heart failure and Crohn's disease, but these are convenient titles simply to slot patients into symptom-relieving categories which do little to reverse the disease process or afford a permanent cure. Symptom-relieving medication postpones the day when major organ failures result. *This is unsustainable medicine.*

My early days in NHS General Practice were exciting. I learned to expect miracles as the norm! I watched a child's 'congenital' deafness resolve on a dairy-free diet; I saw patients with years of headaches see relief from cutting out gluten-containing grains; I saw women with chronic cystitis gain relief from cutting yeast and sugar from their diets. A proper diagnosis establishing causation has obvious implications for management and potential for cure. What was so astonishing to me was that when I tried to communicate my excitement and experiences to fellow doctors they could not have been less interested and dismissed me as a 'flaky quack'!

However, the greatest challenge came from seeing and treating patients with chronic fatigue syndrome (CFS/ME) (explored in my book *Diagnosis and Treatment of Chronic Fatigue Syndrome*). This was – and still is – the elephant in the room. There was absolutely no doubt that these patients were seriously physically unwell. I saw Olympic athletes, England footballers and cricketers, university lecturers, airline pilots, tough farmers, fire fighters and Gulf War veterans reduced to a life of dependency by debilitating pathological fatigue.

Over time I concluded that I would never be able to write a book about what really helped my patients because it would be out of date as soon as it had been written. However, I now believe that although I do not know, and will never know, all the answers, I do at least have sight of most of the elephant. At least I am asking the right questions and have a chance of recognising some of the answers when they present.

> *. . . dans les champs de l'observation, le hasard ne favorise que les esprits prepares. (In the field of observation, chance favours only the prepared mind.*
>
> LOUIS PASTEUR (1822–1895)

In this book I hope to paint a recognisable picture that will both deliver the intellectual imperative and reasoning behind my ideas and also inspire readers to make the difficult lifestyle changes that will result in long-term good health. But the devil is in the detail – and the detail can be accessed at my website (drmyhill.co.uk), which in the last three years has received over six million hits. This will be constantly updated as I learn more.

What has been so unexpected is that the answers to treating CFS/ME have shed a whole new light on other common medical problems such as cancer, heart disease, dementia and other such degenerative conditions. What follows in this book is a blueprint for good health for all your life. It is the end result of 30 years of trial and error, largely the latter. I hope I am working towards the 'bleedin' obvious'.

I'm not young enough to know it all.

OSCAR WILDE (1854–1900)

How this book is organised

Since we can no longer rely on the medical profession to guide us to a healthy lifestyle we must do it ourselves. This can be achieved only by a true understanding of the underlying mechanisms by which Western diets and lifestyles impact health and create disease.

The idea of this book is to empower people to heal themselves through addressing the root causes of their diseases. (If doctors also find it helpful in improving the health of their patients, I will be doubly gratified.) I hope that what follows is a logical progression from symptoms to identifying the underlying mechanisms, and the relevant interventions, tests and tools with which to tackle the root cause of those symptoms. This is how any garage mechanic would fix a car – first ask the driver what appeared to be wrong with the vehicle (symptoms) and then have a look for tell-tale signs to obtain a working diagnosis. Having established the mechanisms by which things are going wrong, the mechanic is in a position to cure.

Of course, the responsible driver does not wait for something to go wrong. By feeding his car the best possible clean fuel and oil, undergoing regular servicing and driving with due care and attention, he will ensure his car motors on for hundreds of thousands of miles. This is disease prevention.

My job as a doctor is to apply good science to the art of healing. It is my duty to provide the necessary information to allow people to live to their full potential through identifying root causes of disease and treating them with logical interventions. In practice this is a two-pronged approach. Initially we have to identify and correct those aspects of modern Western lifestyles that are so damaging to health. The big issues are diet and nutrition, sleep, exercise, pollution and infection avoidance. Ideally we should all put in place interventions now, before symptoms appear and before these problems trigger pathology.

Preventative interventions include:

1. Paleo-ketogenic diet (staple foods: meat, fish, eggs, vegetables, nuts, seeds, salad, berries; occasional treats: dairy, grains, fruit)
2. Multivitamins, minerals, essential fatty acids

3. Sleep
4. Exercise
5. Sunshine and light
6. Reduction of the chemical burden
7. Sufficient physical and mental security to satisfy our universal need to love and care, and be loved and cared for
8. Avoiding infections and treating these aggressively

These eight measures are what I call the 'Basic Package' and these should be applied in all cases regardless of the current state of health of the individual concerned.

However, none of us lives the perfect life. It is like the old Irish joke – when the traveller asked the way to Dublin, he was told by the local, 'If I were you I wouldn't be starting from here!' We do not seek medical help until we have a problem. So this book will start with symptoms because it is through having those, and a desire to regain our well-being, that we find the strength to put in place the difficult dietary and lifestyle regimes to restore full health.

What this means in practice is that not only is the Basic Package required but also so are the 'Bolt-on Extras' which tackle established symptoms or pathologies. So the last section of this book starts from a disease perspective, revises what has gone before and details the tricks of the trade that have evolved proven and safe techniques.

For the sake of brevity, this guide does not linger on the fine detail. This book then is an introduction, a starting place and, perhaps most importantly, a signpost for those patients who wish to take control of their own health. To do otherwise than this, and to try and write a book which covered every situation for every patient, would make for a dull old read. Furthermore, with experience my ideas and advice will not stand still and so the fine detail of such a book, were it attempted, would need constant updating. I make no apology for this state of affairs as, being old and female, I'm allowed to change my mind!

Whistle-blowing on 21st-century medical practice

Doctors are dangerous. In the United States, healthcare-system-induced deaths are the third leading cause of death after heart disease and cancer.*[2] When doctors go on strike, death rates fall, and when they return to work, death rates rise.[3] However, this effect pales into insignificance when compared with the intellectual neglect demonstrated by doctors failing to understand, recognise and prevent the two major causes of death – namely, heart disease and cancer. The worst example of this neglect is the nonsense propagated by doctors that a high-fat diet results in high cholesterol and consequently in heart and arterial disease – indeed, this has become the popular accepted wisdom. Yet it is completely wrong! It is sugar, fruit sugar, refined carbohydrates and grains that are driving the epidemics of arterial disease, heart disease and cancer. The failure of the medical profession to recognise and act on this is a crime against humanity.

These collective failures mean that it is more dangerous to follow your doctor's advice on diet and take symptom-suppressing medication than to smoke 20 cigarettes a day.

The greatest modern health hazard is metabolic syndrome. This is the clinical picture that results from Western diets and lifestyles. It is easy to diagnose – simply look in the supermarket trolley. If it is largely composed of bread, cereals, biscuits, pasta, fruits, crisps, sweets, chocolate and alcohol then

---

* According to several research studies in the 1990s, a total of 225,000 Americans per year have died as a result of their medical treatments:

   12,000 deaths per year due to unnecessary surgery
   7,000 deaths per year due to medication errors in hospitals
   20,000 deaths per year due to other errors in hospitals
   80,000 deaths per year due to infections in hospitals
   106,000 deaths per year due to negative effects of drugs

its owner, and his/her family, has metabolic syndrome. The early symptoms include having to eat very often, not being satisfied with a meat and vegetable meal until a sweet pudding has been eaten, having to snack regularly and eating or drinking to relieve stress. Fatigue, mood swings and insomnia follow. Doctors get involved when these apple-shaped people are found to have high blood pressure and high cholesterol. There follows an inevitable progression to diabetes, heart disease and cancer. We now know arthritis and osteoporosis are long-term effects of metabolic syndrome. Alzheimer's disease too – this has been renamed 'type III diabetes'.

Most doctors have no grasp of the above progression. They fail to appreciate that carbohydrates are eaten in an addictive way. The intellectually risible 'food pyramid' (which places carbohydrates at the bottom as staple foods, with meat and eggs at the top as occasional extras), is evolutionarily incorrect and upside down. Symptom-suppressing drugs and lack of attention to causation together accelerate the underlying degeneration; people become patients on the slippery downhill slope to disease and death. It is entirely predictable that the National Health Service will become overwhelmed.

The British National Health Service is a wonderful institution, with laudable aims and excellent resources. It is staffed by lions but led by intellectual donkeys. These donkeys are the drug-prescribing doctors who fail to identify the root causes of disease. Instead of even attempting to make a proper diagnosis, they simply prescribe symptom-suppressing drugs. We experience symptoms for good reasons – they protect the body from damage. Symptom-suppressing drugs allow us to function but do so at the expense of accelerating the underlying disease process. Pain-killing drugs mean joints are damaged faster and so surgery to replace joints is required sooner.[4] Symptom suppression and accelerated damage result in a snowballing effect of disease, and so more drugs are needed to suppress side-effects. As just one example – acid-blockers to suppress gut symptoms relieve the discomfort but result in low stomach acid, which is a major risk factor for osteoporosis and stomach cancer.

Someone with a stone in their shoe would feel the pain and remove the stone. By contrast a doctor would first prescribe a pain killer to restore normal walking. However, the stone would erode the foot and infection would follow – so an antibiotic would be prescribed. Infection rarely clears where there is a foreign body and so gangrene would ensue, followed by amputation. Crutches or a wheelchair would be prescribed. The dignified, independent person would become a dependant patient facing long-term disability and premature death.

Again, the treatment of asthma has switched what was once a benign, self-limiting condition to a life-long pathology requiring life-long, symptom-suppressing medication. Indeed, when asthma is poorly managed, patients die. Conventional treatment means first the blue inhaler, next the brown inhaler, then both. No thought is given to the causes of asthma, which may be allergy (to foods, inhalants or chemicals), pollution or hyperventilation.

If symptom-suppressing drugs are ineffective, then a further line of defence is to blame the patient. Psychiatrists call this 'somatisation' – people are imagining their symptoms. This is a highly successful method of preventing these patients from ever returning to that 'diagnosing'' doctor again because the patient, quite rightly, loses faith in the doctor's abilities and looks elsewhere for answers. However, from the doctor's perspective, they (usually) never see this patient again and so they wrongly assume that their 'diagnosis' of somatisation has satisfied the patient. The doctor is left with the false impression that the patient is cured and pats himself on the back for a job well done. Worse than this though is what happens if the patient persists, returns to the doctor and does not accept the somatisation 'diagnosis'. In that case, the patient is blamed, once again, but this time for being a 'difficult' patient, or even for having views which are resistant to the 'cure' being offered. The phrase 'false illness beliefs' is a common one which is then thrown at such patients. Nowhere is this more apparent than in the treatment of chronic fatigue syndrome – my area of special interest. This was the subject of my first book – *Diagnosis and Treatment of Chronic Fatigue Syndrome - it's mitochondria, not hypochondria*. The complete failure of doctors to identify and treat the underlying physical causes of this condition is a disgrace to the medical profession. It has dehumanised hundreds of thousands of potentially healthy people and consigned them to a life of misery.

The undergraduate and postgraduate education of doctors converts intelligent, motivated, caring teenagers into unquestioning, narrow-minded, one-size-fits-all doctors. These young people have all these fine attributes 'educated' out of them. Medical education is a brain-washing process which stupefies and petrifies the ability of the individual doctor to think independently. These disciplined minds become blinkered to see only avenues of treatment as laid down by the pharmaceutical symptom-suppressing approach. The job of the doctor is to understand the science of the body and convert this 'raw knowledge' to the art of treating individual patients, each of whom has a unique constitution that requires a tailored approach. Indeed, this is where the challenge, the pleasure and the fun of medicine lie. Nothing is so rewarding as the grateful patient whose health has been restored; health is like money –you don't know you've got it until you've lost it!

Drug companies were launched on the back of antibiotics – miraculous life-saving magic bullets which have saved millions of lives. This led to a general belief, happily adopted by the population, that all ills could be dealt with by pills. Symptom-suppressing drugs were found to bring immediate relief of pain, fever and misery. Massive drug company profits ensued. In modern Western society, money trumps truth. The drug companies used their new-found wealth to capture the intellectual and moral high ground through manipulation of drug trials. Either such trials were set up to achieve a desired outcome or adverse outcomes were not published. Doctors achieve academic success and promotion through drug company bank-rolled research – often the drug company reps ghostwrite the academic papers. If doctors fail to conform to the above expectations, they risk loss of job and status.

Doctors who fail to toe the drug-industry-driven, conventional-medicine, symptom-suppressing line are singled out for special attention by the Establishment. Dr David Healy was the subject of professional opprobrium when he flagged up how SSRI antidepressants could trigger suicidal and violent behaviour in some patients. Dr Wendy Savage, in the 1980s, was a pioneer in working to abolish the sausage-machine process of childbirth, where women were not permitted any say in how their babies would be delivered. She suffered at the hands of jealous colleagues who saw their institutions threatened – she was suspended from her job and suffered years of prosecution until she fought back successfully to reinstatement. Dr Rita Pal whistle-blew on North Staffordshire Health Authority a decade before it was found guilty of gross neglect of elderly patients. She was struck off the Medical Register by the General Medical Council as a result of her honesty and integrity. I too have faced 11 years of GMC prosecution and 7 GMC hearings simply because my ideas on medicine lay outside conventional medical practice – at least I have to be thankful that I live in the twenty-first century; earlier heretics were burnt at the stake!

Conventional medicine increasingly is being bypassed by intelligent patients who wish to understand the underlying patho-physiological mechanisms which are causing their ill health. Indeed, I often find myself writing the diagnosis of 'PMITD' in the margin of my clinical notes ('patient more intelligent than doctor').

In addressing these issues in this book, I am whistle-blowing on current medical practice. This Emperor has no clothes.

A child cries out, 'But he isn't wearing anything at all!'
HANS CHRISTIAN ANDERSEN (1805–1875)

CHAPTER 1

Symptoms

– our early warning systems which protect us from invaders and from ourselves

In this chapter I cover the following areas:
1. Symptoms – our early warning system
2. Fatigue – the symptom that arises when energy demand exceeds energy delivery
3. Symptoms that arise from poor energy balance
4. Pathology that arises if poor energy balance symptoms are ignored or masked
5. Pain – not all pain is bad: some is necessary to remain physically fit and well
6. Inflammation symptoms: infection, allergy, autoimmunity
7. Toxic symptoms – usually head/foggy brain, depression, psychosis
8. Deficiency symptoms
9. Hormonal deficiencies

Remember: The detective work starts with symptoms.

1. Symptoms – our early warning system

The best clinical clues come from symptoms and 90 per cent of the diagnosis comes from the patient's history. The commonest symptoms are pain and fatigue.

Symptoms are desirable and therapeutic

These two symptoms, pain and fatigue, are essential to protect us from ourselves. We all experience these symptoms on a daily basis – they tell us what we can and cannot do. Without these warning symptoms we would keep going until we dropped, either because the energy delivery ran out (so the heart and brain would stop) or because we would wear out (healing and repair occur during sleep and rest). We ignore or suppress these symptoms at our peril.

Many other symptoms arise downstream of these two most common issues. This happens because we ignore the early warning signs that pain and fatigue represent, or interfere with them, or try to suppress them. Often pathology arises as a result of adopting this 'ignore, interfere and suppress' type of medicine.

For this reason, symptoms should always prompt us to ask the question 'Why?' Collections of symptoms may provide further clues as to causation.

2. Fatigue – the symptom that arises when energy demand exceeds energy delivery

> *Annual income twenty pounds, annual expenditure nineteen pounds*
> *nineteen and six, result happiness. Annual income twenty pounds,*
> *annual expenditure twenty pounds ought and six, result misery.*
>
> Mr Micawber from *David Copperfield*,
> CHARLES DICKENS (1812–1870)

Fatigue is the symptom that arises when energy demand exceeds energy delivery. This means there should be a two-pronged approach to treating fatigue – improve energy delivery systems and identify mechanisms by which energy is wasted.

3. Symptoms that arise from poor energy balance

The symptoms that arise from poor energy balance may be described as 'mild' or 'severe' and the following checklists can be used as a rule of thumb to decide where you are on the generalised fatigue scale.

Mild symptoms

The patient will:
- Become an owl – won't be able to get up in the mornings, sleeps in at weekends.
- Start to use addictions to cope with fatigue – especially caffeine, sugar and refined carbohydrates.
- Have to consciously pace activity – and look forward to rest time and sleep.
- Dread Monday mornings, if in employment.
- Lose the ability (or it will become an effort) to enjoy himself.
- Treasure 'chill out' time in the evenings.

- Lose usual stamina – will not be able to achieve normal levels of fitness.
- Experience a decline in muscular strength.
- Become irritable, experience mild anxiety and low mood – these symptoms are imposed by the brain to prevent us spending energy frivolously. Having fun means spending energy.
- Feel mildly stressed – this symptom of stress arises when the brain knows it does not have the energy reserves to deal with physical, emotional and mental demands.
- Experience joint and muscle stiffness – for tissues to slide over each other with minimal friction requires them to be at just the right temperature. Poor energy delivery means the body runs colder.

These symptoms are often seen as part of the ageing process. This is because mitochondria, which are the engines of cells that generate energy, are also responsible for the ageing process. Numbers of mitochondria fall with age. So as we age we have to pace our activities. This is because our body's ability to generate energy reduces hand in hand with the falling numbers of mitochondria. The obvious corollary is: look after the mitochondria and slow down the ageing process.

Energy **delivery** is all about the **collective** functioning of mitochondria, the thyroid gland, the adrenal glands, the liver, the gut, the heart and the lungs, along with the all-important diet. Together these are responsible for producing the energy molecule ATP (adenotriphosphate). ATP is the currency of energy in the body and a molecule of ATP can buy any job, from muscle contraction to a nerve impulse, or from hormone synthesis to immune activity. Without ATP none such is possible.

Severe symptoms

The patient will experience:

Poor stamina – One molecule of ATP is converted to ADP (adenodiphosphate) and recycled back to ATP via mitochondria every 10 seconds. If this recycling is slow, then poor stamina (mental and physical) and muscle weakness will result very quickly.

Pain – If you run out of ATP because mitochondria cannot keep up with demand, then there is a switch into anaerobic metabolism with the production of lactic acid. One molecule of glucose, burned aerobically in mitochondria, can produce 32–36 molecules of ATP (depending on efficiency). Anaerobic production generates just two molecules of ATP together with one molecule of lactic acid. It is very inefficient. Furthermore, to clear the lactic acid requires six molecules of ATP. This is a particular problem for my CFS patients who simply do not have the energy reserves to clear the lactic acid and therefore suffer prolonged lactic acid burn. When this occurs in the heart, patients are told they have 'atypical chest pain', whereas what they are actually experiencing is angina.

Slow recovery from exertion and delayed fatigue – As ATP is drained, the body can employ another metabolic trick. Two molecules of ADP (that is, two phosphates) combine to form one molecule of ATP (three phosphates) and one of AMP (adenomonophosphate – that is, one phosphate). This is called the 'adenylate kinase' reaction. The good news is that we have another molecule of ATP. The bad news is that AMP is poorly recycled and drains out of the system. The body then has to make brand new ATP. It can do this from a sugar molecule, but this involves a complex and time-consuming piece of biochemistry – the 'pentose phosphate shunt'. Thus there is delayed fatigue. This symptom is one that characterises the clinical picture of pathological fatigue (that is, CFS) because more severe tissue damage starts to occur at this point of very poor energy delivery.

Foggy brain – The brain is greatly demanding of energy. At rest it consumes 20 per cent of the total energy generated in the body. Poor energy delivery results in foggy brain, poor short-term memory and difficulty multi-tasking and problem solving.

Dizzy spells – These too are symptomatic of the brain running out of energy. This is commonly due to low blood pressure or blood sugar levels suddenly dropping.

Very low mood and depression – ATP multi-tasks! It is not just the energy molecule but also a neurotransmitter in its own right. To be precise, it is a co-transmitter – neurotransmitters such as dopamine, GABA, serotonin and acetylcholine do not work unless ATP is present. Disorders of mood such as anxiety and depression would be much better treated if energy delivery issues were tackled.

Anxiety and the feeling of severe stress – These feelings arise because sufferers know they do not have the energy to deal with expected and unexpected demands. Anxiety creates another vicious cycle because this kicks an emotional hole in the energy bucket and interferes with sleep.

Low cardiac output – The heart is a pump which again demands energy. If ATP is not freely available, then it cannot pump powerfully. Weak beats result in poor circulation. The heart tries to compensate by beating faster, but this too is energy demanding. Energy delivery cannot keep up and so blood pressure falls precipitously. Clinically this means my severe CFS patients cannot stand for long, or sometimes even short, periods of time. These patients often have to lie down. Rest is much more restful if we lie down! In addition, there is a vicious cycle present here. Low cardiac output compounds all the above problems of poor energy delivery because during periods of low cardiac output, fuel and oxygen delivery are additionally impaired. So mitochondria go slow simply because they do not have the raw materials to function well. This is just one of the many vicious cycles I see in CFS.

Intolerance of cold – No engine works with 100 per cent efficiency. Some energy is always lost as heat and this helps to keep us warm. Core temperature is often recognised as a particular symptom of hypothyroidism, but it is actually a symptom of poor energy delivery of which hypothyroidism is a part. Being cold results in another vicious cycle – enzymes need heat; roughly speaking a 10 degree rise in temperature doubles their rate of reaction. Being cold means that mitochondrial enzymes, thyroid enzymes and adrenal enzymes, all essential for function, will run slow.

Intolerance of heat – One method of heat control is to pump blood to the skin. The skin is the largest organ of the body and pumping blood round the skin increases cardiac output by 20 per cent. This explains why we all fatigue more quickly on hot days and why exposure to high levels of heat is unsustainable for my severe CFS patients.

Variable blurred vision – The muscles of the eye are energy demanding and so if energy delivery is poor, CFS patients will be unable to contract eye muscles to allow the lens to focus.

Light intolerance – The retina, weight for weight, is the most energy-demanding organ of the body. It consumes energy 100 times faster than the rest of the body. This is because the business of converting a light signal into an electrical signal requires massive amounts of ATP. Light intolerance is a feature of severe CFS. It is also a feature of migraine which, I suspect, also has energy delivery as one possible cause. We cannot generate energy without producing free radicals, and these damage tissues. I suspect this explains the high incidence of eye pathology with ageing, such as cataracts, glaucoma and macular degeneration.

Noise intolerance – Again, the business of converting vibrations of air and bone molecules into an electrical signal for the brain to interpret is greatly demanding of energy.

Shortness of breath – If energy delivery at the cellular level is impaired, the brain may misinterpret this as poor oxygen delivery and stimulate the respiratory centre to breathe harder. This may result in hyperventilation which actually makes the situation worse. Hyperventilation changes the acidity of the blood so oxygen sticks more avidly to haemoglobin, thus worsening oxygen delivery. Shortness of breath may also result from heart failure, respiratory distress and anaemia.

Susceptibility to infection – The immune system is greatly demanding of energy and of raw materials such as zinc, vitamin C and selenium. A common cause of this symptom is also hypochlorrhydria because we need an acid stomach to absorb minerals.

Loss of libido – This makes perfect biological sense – procreation and raising children requires large amounts of energy.

4. Pathology that arises if poor energy balance symptoms are ignored or masked

Organ damage and organ failure arise as a result of ignoring or masking poor energy balance symptoms.

Heart failure – Symptoms usually come before organ damage, but not always. The kidney, for example, suffers in silence. However, if symptoms are ignored, then organ damage will result. Fatigue is the symptom that arises when energy demand exceeds energy delivery, and when this occurs at the cellular level, levels of ATP (the energy molecule) within cells will fall. If levels of ATP fall below a critical amount, this triggers cell apoptosis – that is, cell suicide. Indeed, this is part of the ageing process – we literally lose cells and our organs slowly shrink. If the situation becomes critical, either because total energy delivery fails or the number of cells declines, we develop organ failure and ultimately die. It is this process which prevents us from living forever. A common organ failure that results in death is heart failure – we are currently seeing an epidemic of heart failure, which I believe partly stems from the prescription of statins. One of the side effects of statins is that they inhibit the body's own production of coenzyme Q10, which is an essential co-factor in normal mitochondrial function. (Interestingly, the benefits of statins seem to have little to do with their effect on cholesterol levels – any benefit appears to arise because biochemically they look like vitamin D. Vitamin D is highly protective against heart disease, cancer and degenerative conditions. Statins are a particular hate of mine.)

Dementia is brain organ failure. Essentially this arises when the speed at which nerves process electrical signals slows down. That process is enormously

demanding of energy. A major cause of dementia is arteriosclerosis, due to
poor oxygen and fuel delivery to the brain. I suspect statins are also partly
responsible for our epidemic of dementia.

Poor immunity – The immune system is enormously demanding of energy
and this probably explains why elderly people are much more likely to die
from infection than younger people, simply because they do not have the
energy to power the immune system to fight infections effectively.

5. Pain

Remember, not all pain is bad: some is necessary to remain physically fit and
well. Pain is the symptom that protects the body from damaging itself. Its function is to make us stop so as to prevent further damage and rest the painful area
so that healing and repair can take place. Leprosy causes digits and limbs to be
lost simply because the condition destroys nerves. The body cannot protect a
numb limb from damage.

Modest amounts of pain are essential for good health. The body is very
efficient – no energy resources are wasted. This has been an essential policy
for evolutionary success – we have to be intrinsically lazy. However, in our
modern world of plenty we become lazy because we can. Pushing the system
(which in Nature occurs at least once a week during a predator-prey interaction) generates pain as a result of lactic acid burn together with mild wear and
tear of muscles, connective tissue and joints. This modest pain is a powerful
stimulus to lay down new tissue with its new complement of mitochondria,
and this increases physical fitness. The difference between weak and strong,
little and large muscles is the number of mitochondria.

Astronauts cannot remain long in space because there is no gravity and no
mechanical stress on bones – they quickly develop osteoporosis and muscle
wasting. Putting a patient to bed is dangerous for the same reasons.

Causes of pain

When taking a history from a patient, I constantly think mechanisms – the idea
is to establish such mechanisms because this has implications for treatment.
The nature of the pain may provide useful clinical clues. Useful categories of
pain include:

Mechanical – In mechanical pain with tissue damage (which may arise additionally from subsequent inflammation), the sensitive coverings of organs

are irritated. The pain from a broken bone comes from the periosteal membrane that covers the bone. The pain of an inflamed or ruptured gut (peritonitis) comes from the peritoneal membrane that wraps round the gut. The meninges covering the brain are highly sensitive and the pain of meningitis is severe. Pleural membranes that surround the lungs when inflamed cause intense pain on breathing – called pleurisy. A feature of these pains is that the patient immobilises the area – any movement makes things much worse. Patients keep the affected area very still because movement is excruciatingly painful.

Muscle spasm from smooth muscle ('unconscious' muscle, such as in the gut, womb and bladder) – This produces some of the most severe pains. Examples include labour pains, renal colic (from stones), gall stone colic (from stones in the gall bladder), bowel colic from wind, constipation, adhesions or other such blockage. These spasms are mechanically caused as the muscles try to move an obstruction. A feature of this pain is that often movement is helpful and the patient is restless. The pain is 'colicky', that is to say the severity waxes and wanes.

Muscle spasm from skeletal muscle is often extremely painful. I suspect this is often misdiagnosed as 'pinched nerve' pain. Often the pain occurs following a minor movement, not enough to cause any damage. It starts suddenly and is described as lancinating, knife-like, sharp or like an electric shock. The sufferer is completely floored. After a few minutes it settles, but any awkward movement may provoke it again. Cramp, stiff neck and 'stiff man syndrome' are examples of acute muscle spasm which may be due to allergic muscles, mineral imbalances, dehydration or acidity.

Lactic acid burn from poor energy delivery – In this event there is a switch into anaerobic metabolism with the production of lactic acid, and this causes pain. It starts with a dull ache and, if not relieved, will continue up to the severe pain of a myocardial infarction requiring morphine for relief. Athletes experience this daily and it allows and limits peak performance – no pain, no gain! Lactic acid burn in the heart is angina. The feature of this pain is that it comes with exercise and is relieved by rest, only to come again with exercise. However, in patients with very poor energy delivery (such as CFS) the lactic acid burn may be very persistent and not recognised as such. The best example comes from CFS patients who develop chest pain – actually this is angina, due not to poor blood supply but to poor mitochondrial function. Acute unremitting lactic acid burn as caused by an arterial obstruction causes severe pain such as that experienced in a myocardial infarction, pulmonary embolus or acute arterial obstruction. I suspect one mechanism of the pain of migraine has to do with poor energy delivery to the brain. Indeed, many of my CFS patients describe chronic headache which I suspect is lactic acid burn in the brain.

Muscle and joint stiffness – This is a common but greatly overlooked cause of discomfort. The tissues do not slide smoothly over each other and the friction results in a sensation of stiffness as the body tries to protect itself from sudden movements. The person has to 'warm up' slowly before attempting action. Inflammation (such as in allergy) may cause this. I suspect that mineral imbalance is also a cause since so many patients respond well to topical magnesium applied to the skin.

Inflammation is nearly always painful, although mild inflammation may present with a lesser pain symptom of itch. Inflammation is characterised by pain, swelling (with the potential for mechanical irritation), heat, redness (due to increased blood flow) and loss of function (as the body protects itself by shutting down that department). Inflammation pains are often described as 'burning' in nature – often worse in the mornings and improving as the day progresses. My patients who have inflammation from silicone implants often describe the pain as burning. 'Throbbing' is a feature of inflammation. Increased pressure makes the pain worse – for example, the person with a severe toothache or sinusitis finds their symptoms are worse when lying down. The symptoms of inflammation may be reduced with cooling and may be worsened by heat.

Inflammatory pain at rest (for example at night) I suspect is healing and repair pain. The body cannot heal and repair unless the organ is rested and shut down. Healing and repair involve the immune system and inflammation.

Nerve pain can be electric shock–like and markedly dependent on position or movement, implying a compression issue. (Anyone who has banged their 'funny bone' (the ulnar nerve at the elbow) will recognise this.) The pain follows the area that the nerve supplies, so a careful mapping of the pain gives useful anatomical clues. Sciatica typically starts in the buttock and radiates down the back of the leg. Carpel tunnel syndrome involves the thumb, index, middle and part of the ring finger, sparing the little finger. It may arise because the nerve is pinched which can be a mechanical problem or because of swelling of soft tissues from inflammation (often due to allergy) or myxoedema (severe underactive thyroid). Tic douloureaux (or trigeminal neuralgia – that is, severe pain in the side of the face) is, I suspect, due to allergic nerves – the mechanism may be similar to allergic muscle: sensitisation due to mechanical or infectious trauma and an inflammation maintained by allergy. This may be allergy to foods, microbes, chemicals and so on.

All pain is perceived more where there is fear, anxiety, depression and loss of hope – the mental and emotional state is critical. That is why it is so important to put the patient in control of the diagnostic process.

Intuition is a wonderful thing. In my experience, the untrained patient often makes a remarkably accurate diagnosis. I always listen very carefully to pain descriptions because this is very helpful in establishing causation.

Listen to your patient, for he will give you the diagnosis . . .

Sir William Osler (1849–1919)

The key to treating pain is not to mask it with pain killers but to ask the question 'why?' before the clinical picture becomes blurred. Once pain has become longstanding and chronic, many of the above mechanisms come into play and it is more difficult to tease out the different strands that need tackling. Other vicious cycles then cut in.

One final point in this section is **malaise**. Many patients struggle to explain this feeling – it is a feeling of not being well. I suspect it reflects low-grade tissue damage and poor energy delivery resulting in low-grade inflammation. This may not show up in standard blood tests. It may be reflected in a cell-free DNA test – this is a measure of cell damage. Malaise is very common in CFS patients who cannot pace their activity because they do not even have enough energy for house-keeping duties (basic gut, liver, kidney, heart, brain, etc function). Some products of inflammation impact directly on the brain resulting in 'illness behaviour' – again this is a protective mechanism to allow rest and protect one from oneself!

6. Inflammation symptoms: infection, allergy, autoimmunity

Inflammation is characterised by the cardinal symptoms of pain, swelling, heat (redness) and loss of function. Think inflammation if there is this combination of symptoms. But this begs the question as to the cause of inflammation. We all know the obvious one – infection. But allergy and autoimmunity also result in inflammation and may cause almost any symptom. Historically, syphilis was said to be 'the great mimic', producing almost any symptom and pathology. This has been replaced by allergy and in the future autoimmunity will be a major player – currently 1 in 20 Westerners has an autoimmune disease (see page 194).

The living organism that we are is potentially a free lunch for others. We fight a constant 'arms race' against invading microbes and parasites. Indeed, it could be argued that all disease processes that involve inflammation are part of this arms race.

Many occasional symptoms exist to physically expel or kill invaders. These same disease processes are invoked where there is allergy. Acute symptoms are most likely to be infectious, with chronic or recurring symptoms being allergic or autoimmune.

Symptoms of acute inflammation

These include:

Fatigue – This is an essential symptom to enforce rest so that the immune system has the energy to fight back.

Malaise and 'illness behaviour' – Men seem much better at this than women (ho ho!).

Fever – Most microbes are killed by heat.

Swollen lymph nodes ('glands').

Mucous and catarrh – These physically wash out microbes.

Runny eyes – Ditto.

Coughing and sneezing – These physically blast out microbes in the airways.

Airways narrowing, wheezing, asthma – This results in the air we breathe becoming more turbulent so microbes are thrown against and stick to the mucous lining of the airways to be coughed up and swallowed and killed by an acid bath of the stomach.

Vomiting – This is an essential defence against food poisoning and microbes that have been inhaled (which are coughed up and swallowed).

Diarrhoea – Ditto.

Colic – Ditto.

Cystitis – Emptying the bladder of urine clears out microbes.

So, for example, look at a hay fever sufferer. Without clinical details, I might diagnose a cold. Looking at an inflamed patch on the skin, without clinical details, I might not be sure if this was allergic eczema, sunburn, chemical burn, infected cellulitis, viral or autoimmune rash! The patient's history is vital.

With acute infection such as 'flu it is potentially dangerous to use symptom-suppressing medication, which interferes with these natural defences. It has the potential to make problems much worse. I would caution against taking symptom-modifying medication which interferes with the body's natural processes of eliminating microbes. Indeed, I suspect this is why we are currently seeing epidemics of post-viral fatigue syndromes.

Allergy and autoimmunity –
consider with more chronic symptoms

Allergy is today's great mimic and can produce any symptom, including all of the above.

Whilst any antigen can cause any symptoms (Dr John Mansfield described a case of osteoarthritis of the hip due to allergy to house dust mite), common things are common. Chronologically, symptoms often start in the nose and throat (ENT) and extend to the gut, brain and then any other organ. If a symptom has become chronic then I would consider the following allergens in order of likelihood:

ENT symptoms such as catarrh, deafness, glue ear, snoring and
> obstructive sleep apnoea, voice changes, cough – Allergy to dairy,
> yeast (fermenting gut).

Tinnitus – Allergy to foods or gut microbes (I suspect this may also
> contribute to age-related deafness – Beethoven went deaf following
> salmonella infection). Caffeine may cause tinnitus by a toxic reaction.

Irritable bowel syndrome – Allergy to foods and upper fermenting
> gut problems.

Inflammatory bowel disease – Ditto.

Asthma – Allergy to foods, biological inhalants and gut microbes.

Headache – Allergy to aspartame or dairy. Caffeine may cause a
> toxic headache.

Migraine – typical allergic headache, but there are other causes, notably
> poor energy delivery and toxic reactions from vaso-active amines.

Eczema and urticaria – Allergy to foods and gut microbes.

Acne and rosacea – Ditto.

Interstitial cystitis, chronic prostatitis/epididymitis, vulvitis –
> Allergy to gut microbes, especially yeast.

Arthritis – Allergy to foods and gut microbes.

Allergic muscles, tendons, connective tissue – Allergy to dairy, gluten
> grains and gut microbes.

Fatigue – Allergy to gluten grains.

Furthermore, one can be allergic to anything under the sun, including the sun. In considering allergy problems, I think of groups of allergens as causes of problems which may be:

• Foods and food additives

- Biological inhalants – house dust mite, pollens, animal danders, moulds and others
- Chemicals – toxic metals, pesticides and volatile organic compounds (perfumes and such) and others
- Microbes in the gut and elsewhere – yeast, bacteria, viruses, parasites, worms and possibly others

The above sensitivities may be worsened by other pro-inflammatory or irritant factors – notably:

- **Electromagnetic radiation** – Electrical sensitivity is a real and growing problem, with adverse reactions possible to mobile phone masts, wi-fi, computers, TVs and so on. It appears the mechanism of this is by activating voltage-gated calcium channels to make membranes more irritable.
- **Noise pollution and infrasound** – Wind turbine syndrome is a real condition with additional problems of amplitude modulation. The mechanism of damage is two-fold: firstly, sleep deprivation; secondly, infrasound sets up resonant frequencies within body cavities causing disturbing symptoms of headache, unease, agitation, vibrations, vertigo and gut disturbances.

7. Toxic symptoms

Food is dangerous stuff. If you look at life from the point of view of a plant, it does not want to be eaten, so it has evolved many poisons to protect it from such. Examples include lectins, alkaloids, alkylating agents (such as glycosides in cycad seeds from Guam that cause motor neurone disease), mycotoxins and so on.

By contrast, meat and meat fat are non-toxic – animals have evolved other systems of defence; they can run away! I suspect the main ways in which meat may be toxic arise from the cooking of meat and fat at high temperatures, which results in toxic trans fats being produced, or the fermentation of protein where there is upper fermenting gut (see page 201); both of these are complications of recent evolutionary changes. When humans learned to cook and to farm, this introduced a new range of toxins as the carbohydrate-based foods that are farmed (grains, potatoes) may be fermented in the upper gut to a range of alcohols, D-lactate, hydrogen sulphide and others.

Humans have evolved a fabulous detoxification system in the gut, liver and blood stream to cope with these natural toxins. However, we are all inevitably exposed to further unnatural toxins (see page 228) from the outside world because it is so polluted. I have yet to do a fat biopsy or test for toxic metals and find a normal result. Many of these toxins cause problems because they may:

- Inhibit energy delivery systems (with all the symptoms that arise from such).
- Act as adjuvants to switch on allergy to other substances, and indeed this is the basis of vaccination. There may be pro-inflammatory effects (such as, from toxic metals [used in vaccines]), organophosphates or diesel particulates (these can switch on sensitivity to pollen).
- Act as an antigen and switch on direct allergy to itself (for example, nickel allergy).
- Block hormone systems – For example, our epidemic of type II diabetes partly results from hormone-receptor blocking with insulin resistance. Bromides, fluorides and toxic metals inhibit thyroid hormone receptors.
- Act as hormone mimics (organochlorines have oestrogen-like effects – they can change the sex of crocodiles).
- Switch on cancer (for example, toxic metals, pesticides, VOCs).
- Switch on prion disorders (for example, toxic metals and organophosphates).

However, some toxins are *directly* toxic. The commonest manifestation of such direct toxic stress is in the brain. These toxins include:

Sugar and refined carbohydrate may result in the fermenting gut; this too may produce hangover-like symptoms
Alcohol – from drinking the stuff; we all feel poisoned with a hangover
Caffeine – too much is toxic
Prescription medication
Drugs of addiction

One potential problem is the 'fermenting brain' as described by Professor Nishihara[5]. His idea here is that microbes, probably from the gut or the outside world, get into the brain and ferment neurotransmitters into amphetamine- and LSD-like chemicals. Clinically, this would present with a huge range of psychiatric and psychological symptoms.

8. Deficiency symptoms

Where there are single gross deficiencies in calories, vitamins, minerals and essential fatty acids, a clear clinical picture emerges. We all know the story of scurvy, with gum disease, infection, neuropathy and death. Gross vitamin B3 deficiency results in the memorable dermatitis, diarrhoea, dementia and death. It is very unusual to see such singular pictures in clinical practice. However, many people are suffering from multiple minor deficiencies of vitamins, minerals and essential fatty acids which present with fatigue (see page 33), pain (see page 222), inflammation (see page 208) and inability to detox efficiently (toxicity symptoms).

9. Hormonal deficiencies

Adrenal hormones and thyroid hormones together with hormones involved in blood sugar control are all part of the body's energy delivery systems and deficiencies would present with the symptoms described on page 122.

Sex hormones are essential for procreation. This is a process greatly demanding of energy and resources. If energy delivery systems are faulty, with deficiencies of essential nutrients together with toxic stresses, then sex hormones will suffer downstream, resulting in multiple symptoms of loss of libido, impotence and infertility, with women additionally suffering PMT and gynaecological problems. As I said at the start of this chapter, remember that the detective work starts with symptoms.

Focusing on symptoms

Symptoms, their chronology and the circumstances which trigger or relieve them, provide important clues as to the biochemical, immunological and hormonal lesions that underlie them. Collections of symptoms to indicate problems are dealt with in the relevant sections ahead. Tests provide useful supporting evidence. Identifying the mechanisms has obvious implications for treatment.

Symptoms are the starting point for any diagnosis. I regard a good patient history as one that includes:

Listening carefully to the patient's account of his/her symptoms – Even the words chosen are illuminating. For example, if the patient says he/she feels 'toxic', 'poisoned' or 'hung-over', he/she may be describing the fermenting gut or a toxic exposure. Patients with problems following silicone implants often describe their muscle pain as 'burning'. Indeed, 'burning pain' points to inflammation.

Establishing the chronology of symptoms in order to work out causation.

Childhood problems and stresses give clues about immune and psychological programming. Chemical toxicity and vaccinations impact on both because many are immune adjuvants and affect neurodevelopment.

Family history – Problems run in families and, indeed, so do answers to problems.

Mitochondria come down the female line, so I often see mother–daughter or mother–son combinations, both with CFS. Mitochondria also determine longevity, so look to your mother for this. Gut flora comes down the female line – we acquire mother's gut-friendly, immune-tagged, safe microbes at the point of birth, possibly in utero.

Problems of the immune system – such as allergy, autoimmunity and cancer – run strongly in families.

What is known already – This includes allergies to foods, biologicals (house-dust mites, animals, pollens, moulds, etc), chemicals (perfume, cleaning agents, cosmetics, etc), metals (nickel and jewellery), microbes (post viral infection syndromes) and electrical sensitivity.

Response to treatments already tried – Some people only feel well taking anti-biotics; this could point to allergy to fermenting bacteria in the gut. Others feel terrible on antibiotics; this could point to allergy to fermenting yeast in the gut.

Diet – It is easy to pick the carbohydrate addicts – they often miss breakfast, graze on carb snacks through the day and supper is their biggest meal. Individuals with gluten allergies tend to use cereals, bread, biscuits, cakes, pasta, pizza, etc as staple foods. Individuals with dairy allergies tend to love all dairy products. (I once had a patient, before I could try anything, inform me that when he died he would like to take a cow to heaven with him. He loved milk, butter, cheese, cream and yoghurt! The diagnosis was easy.)

Drinks – I always ask about drinks and how much of them is drunk. These are often high carb, with fruit sugars, artificial sweeteners and other such. Those containing caffeine or alcohol are diuretic. An alcoholic is one who drinks more than his doctor!

Environmental exposures – Foreign travel, sexually transmitted diseases, food poisoning and vaccinations may all switch on inflammation.

Occupational exposures – These may include pesticides (farmers, fumiga-tors, gardeners, pilots and cabin crew, vets, etc); toxic metals (deodorants, jewellery, dental amalgam, etc); volatile organic compounds, or 'VOCs' (polluting industry, air fresheners and cleaners, vehicle fumes, central heat-ing and cookers, smokers/smoking, aerotoxic syndrome, etc).

As a doctor who spends her life talking to patients, I am good at pattern recognition in order to identify the underlying mechanisms that have resulted in the clinical picture that sits in front of me. However, everyone is an expert in their own bodies and minds and, given the right clues, can work out these mechanisms themselves. That is the point of this book.

Having used symptoms to come to a working diagnosis, we then need to put that to the test using appropriate investigations, choosing the relevant tools to treat and, most importantly, assessing the response to treatment.

CHAPTER 2

Mechanisms and tests

– the mechanisms by which symptoms and diseases are produced and tests with which to identify those mechanisms

It is now time to consider the all-important 'energy equation': energy delivery minus energy expenditure. It is apposite here to quote again the 'Micawber Principle':

> *Annual income twenty pounds, annual expenditure nineteen pounds*
> *nineteen and six, result happiness. Annual income twenty pounds,*
> *annual expenditure twenty pounds nought and six, result misery.*

> Mr Micawber in *David Copperfield*
> Charles Dickens (1812–1870)

So it is with energy as it is with money!

First, consider the mechanisms of energy delivery, which can be likened to the various functional parts, or indeed servicing, of the internal combustion engine. These functional parts all play vital, but different, roles in converting the chemical energy, the fuel in the petrol tank, to kinetic energy, the desired motion of the vehicle. So it is with humans also, with the desired outcomes being not only motion but also brain function, immune function, cell repair and growth and so on. All of these individual and crucial roles will be discussed in detail later on in this part of the book, but for now, it is enough to list the internal combustion engine functional parts and their corresponding human analogies:

A. Mechanisms of energy delivery

1. Fuel in the tank	Diet, hypoglycaemia, micronutrients and gut function
2. Regular servicing	Sleep
3. The engine	Mitochondria
4. Oxygen and fuel delivery	Heart, lung, blood supply
5. Accelerator pedal	Thyroid gland
6. Gear box	Adrenal gland
7. Exhaust system	Liver, kidney, detoxing
8. The driver of the car	The brain

Next consider the mechanisms of energy expenditure. Here, focus is placed on those pathological mechanisms which result in energy being wasted, rather than the 'housekeeping' energy expenditure which the body is required to do on a daily basis – for example, basic metabolism, physical and mental work. Once again these areas will be covered in detail later on, but for now it suffices to list the generalised headings:

B. Mechanisms of energy expenditure

NORMAL ENERGY EXPENDITURE:
1. Housekeeping duties – basic metabolism:
   heart, gut, liver, kidney, lung, hormonal function
2. Physical activity
3. Mental activity

WASTEFUL ENERGY EXPENDITURE:
1. Immunological holes:
   a. Inflammation for healing and repair
   b. Inflammation in infection
   c. Useless inflammation in allergy
      and autoimmunity
2. Emotional holes

C. Mechanisms of mechanical damage

1. Structure, friction and wear and tear
2. Allergic joints, connective tissue and muscles

Acid-alkali balance

Many of the above problems are worsened if the body is too acidic. This is an inevitable part of Western diets because carbohydrates are fermented in the gut to leave an acid residue. This may result in a metabolic acidosis which can be diagnosed from simple blood tests. If one totals the sodium plus potassium and takes away the chloride and bicarbonate (for the mathematicians this is $(Na + K) - (Cl + HCO_3)$) this leaves a figure which should be less than 14 mE/l. This is called the 'anion gap'. If the figure is higher, this means there is a metabolic acidosis. This can be treated with magnesium carbonate 1–3 grams taken at night (or at least 90 minutes after food). Indeed, many cases of arthritis, including gout, can be greatly improved by this simple intervention. See www.drmyhill.co.uk/wiki/Acid-Alkali_balance.

D. Growth promotion

- Benign tumours
- Cancer
- Prion disorders – Alzheimer's, Parkinson's disease, CJD, possibly motor neurone disease

E. Genetic mechanisms

However, before embarking upon detailed accounts of all these types of energy delivery and energy expenditure mechanisms, and the other issues mentioned above, it is wise to spend a little time discussing the general approach to diagnosis.

The general approach to diagnosis

I use the patient's clinical history, symptoms, signs and family history to make a working diagnosis. This diagnosis is based on identifying the underlying mechanisms by which things can go wrong because this has obvious implications for management. Tests are very helpful to confirm or refute a diagnosis. Unfortunately, we do not have a complete range of tests to identify all possible mechanisms – tests for allergy, for example, are notoriously unreliable. My role is to interpose myself between the Science and the patient. Medicine is still an Art! We have to use the combined acumen of doctor, patient and laboratory to deliver a result and make it work for the individual patient – and every patient is unique.

- Firstly we must identify problems of energy delivery so as to be able to make the pot of energy that is available on a daily basis as large as possible.
- Secondly we have to identify how that energy is being spent.

Energy is essential for 'housekeeping duties' (that is, basic metabolism), for physical work and for mental work. Indeed, two thirds of all energy spent in the body goes on these house-keeping duties. Many of my CFS patients do not even have sufficient energy for these house-keeping duties and so there is none to spare for physical and mental activity. We all have to pace our activity to match daily demands. The problem is that spending energy, like spending money, is fun! We have to be disciplined. Clinically, I see two common 'holes' in that energy pot when energy is being spent uselessly or even destructively. These are the emotional hole and the immunological hole.

So we maximise the pot and minimise the holes.

Maximising the pot

The body works like an engine and is amenable to the same logical approach. Going back to my car analogy at the start of the chapter, in order of clinical prevalence I consider the following issues:

Fuel in the tank	Diet (macronutrients and micronutrients), hypoglycaemia and raw materials and gut function
Regular servicing	Sleep
Engine of the car	Mitochondria
Oxygen supply	Blood supply
Accelerator pedal	Thyroid gland
Gear box	Adrenal gland
Exhaust system	Liver, kidney, detoxing
Driver	Brain
Structure	Muscle, connective tissue, bone

Perhaps the single most important aspect, and the most overlooked of the above, are the mitochondria. These organelles (structures within our cells) have become my special area of interest. Mitochondria determine how much energy we have available on a daily basis; they determine the ageing process and we now know that most diseases, from cancer and diabetes to autism and dementia, have mitochondrial pathology.

Look after your mitochondria and they will look after you.

Minimising the holes

Basic metabolism – that is, what I have called 'housekeeping duties' – is unavoidable but essential. It consumes about two thirds of all energy production. This is to keep the gut, liver, kidneys, bone marrow, heart, lungs, glands, brain and so on ticking over just to stay alive. It happens unconsciously and we are not aware of energy being spent in these departments. The areas over which we do have control, or we can manage, are:

Mental work – the brain weighs 2 per cent of body weight but
  consumes 20 per cent of total energy production
Physical work
Immunological holes
Inflammation for healing and repair
Inflammation in infection
Useless inflammation in allergy and autoimmunity
Emotional holes
Mechanical damage: structure, friction and wear and tear
Genetics

The first two of these (mental and physical activity) can be regulated by 'pacing', and the others are dealt with in detail in what follows. Now we are ready to move onto the nuts and bolts of the energy delivery and expenditure mechanisms.

A. Mechanisms of energy delivery

1. Fuel in the tank

The most important feature of the 'fuel in the tank' is diet.

> Let food be thy medicine and medicine be thy food.
>
> HIPPOCRATES, the father of Western medicine (c. 460–370 BC)

Paleo-ketogenic diet

Humans, and indeed all mammals, evolved over millions of years eating a Paleo-ketogenic diet based on protein, fat and vegetable fibre. Even vegetarian mammals who rely on vegetable fibre power themselves with fat – the vegetable fibre is fermented to short-chain fatty acids in the gut.

The human brain was able to grow in size and complexity quickly because primitive man hunted meat, fished and gathered shell fish. Meat and fat provide the perfect raw materials for brain structure and function, together with the necessary stimuli for growth through social cooperation for successful hunting. There may have been the occasional carbohydrate bonanza as the banana tree ripened, but this would have been relatively short lived. Fossilised human turds look like dog turds! Primitive man was primarily a carnivore. Cave paintings show hunters.

Fat is a wonderful fuel. It is energy dense, is not fermented in the gut and is easily utilised. So the human gut shrank. This made man a much more successful hunter because he was not carrying around a huge fermenting belly. Indeed, the human stomach, small intestine, caecum and colon, vast in vegetable-fibre fermenters, have shrunk compared to our ancestors. The human appendix is an evolutionary remnant. It is only in the last few thousand years – negligible in evolutionary time – that starchy carbohydrates have crept into the diet as man has learned to farm and to cook. It is only in the past few decades that sugar and refined carbohydrates have replaced fat as our main fuel, with disastrous metabolic consequences. Since the Neolithic, or Agricultural, revolution, human brain sizes have decreased by 8 per cent. Even now through their lives, vegetarians suffer much more brain shrinkage than meat eaters; vegans even more.

> *Fat is the most valuable food known to man.*
> Professor John Yudkin (1910–1995)

I recommend all my patients read the excellent presentation by Barry Groves (author of *Trick and Treat, Homo carnivorus*, which can be found at: files .meetup.com/1463924/Homo%20Carnivorous-WAPF2.pdf.

For many, a good understanding of the evolutionary imperatives is enough to make them change their diet.

Some vegetable fibre is still essential to nourish the lining of the large bowel. This is dependent for its fuel source on the fermentation of vegetable fibre by friendly anaerobic microbes – namely, 'bacteroides'. Complete lack of bacteroides may result in major pathology, such as ulcerative colitis.

Fruit would have been consumed only once a year when the fruit tree ripened. Modern fruits are different – carefully bred to appeal to modern man's addictive sweet tooth. Primitive man's idea of an apple would have been a crab apple!

There may have been, as noted, the occasional carbohydrate bonanza, and so perhaps metabolic syndrome (see page 213) evolved as a mechanism to store these carbohydrates as liver glycogen and fats. Female sex hormones do the same to lay down fat in preparation for the energy-sapping business of pregnancy and breast feeding. However, primitive man soon reverted to his primitive low-carb diet by contrast with modern Westerners, who are in a permanent state of carb addiction, leading to metabolic syndrome and the serious diseases that result therefrom, especially diabetes.

Some people may have adapted to cope with the relatively recent addition of unrefined carbohydrates to our diet, but I suspect not many, with the numbers who can do so declining with age. I know my CFS patients are carnivorous evolutionary relics – they have not adapted. I do not have CFS but I too function much better eating a Paleo-ketogenic diet. There are many interventions I can suggest which are clinically helpful, but in the treatment of almost any patient, a good Paleo-ketogenic diet is nearly always the single most important and most difficult intervention required. I spend more time talking about diet than all other interventions put together. In particular then, it is important to look in detail at carbohydrate intolerance and hypoglycaemia, the next sub-section of this 'fuel in the tank' section.

Carbohydrate intolerance and hypoglycaemia – the major cause of ill health in Westerners

The petrol for our mitochondrial engines (the energy factories within our cells) is ultimately what are known as 'acetate groups'. Evolution intended that these come from, in order of importance, three possible sources:

1. beta oxidation of fat
2. glycogen stores in the liver and muscle
3. short-chain fatty acids from the fermentation of vegetable fibre in the large bowel

The problem with eating sugar, fruit sugar and refined carbohydrate is that these primary fuel-delivery systems are bypassed. This is dangerous metabolism.

It is critically important for the body to maintain blood sugar levels within a narrow range. Sugar is petrol, essential but highly toxic stuff. If blood sugar levels fall too low, energy supply to all tissues, particularly the brain, is impaired. However, if blood sugar levels rise too high, then this is very damaging to arteries, and the long-term effect of arterial disease is heart disease and stroke. This is caused by sugar sticking to proteins and fats to make AGEs (advanced glycation end products), which accelerate the ageing process. Glycosylated haemoglobin, or HbA1c, is just one such AGE. Poorly controlled diabetics have high levels of AGEs and are at high risk of disease and death.

Excess sugar flooding into the system after a high-carbohydrate meal should be mopped up by the muscle and liver glycogen sponge (see page 206), but only so long as there is space there for both muscle and liver to act in this way. The sponge empties when we exercise. Exercise depletes glycogen in the muscles, so squeezing the sponge dry. This system of control works perfectly well until it is upset by eating excessive carbohydrate or not exercising. Eating excessive sugar at one meal – or excessive refined carbohydrate, which is rapidly digested into sugar – can suddenly overwhelm the muscle and liver's normal glycogen sponge control of blood sugar levels.

Sugar and refined carbohydrates are a particular problem for my CFS patients because they do not have the energy to create a metabolic glycogen sponge.

As I have said, humans evolved over millions of years eating a diet that was very low in sugar and had no refined carbohydrate. Control of blood sugar therefore largely occurred as a result of eating this Paleo-ketogenic diet and the fact that we were exercising vigorously, so any excessive sugar in the blood was mopped up by the glycogen sponge. Nowadays, the situation is different: we eat large amounts of sugar and refined carbohydrate and do not exercise enough to squeeze dry the glycogen sponge. The body therefore has to cope with this excessive sugar load by other mechanisms.

The key player here is insulin, a hormone excreted by the pancreas. This is effective at bringing blood sugar levels down and does so by eventually shunting the sugar into fat. The amount of insulin released is proportional to the rate at which blood sugars rise – this is what makes dietary sugar so pernicious; it is rapidly absorbed and levels in the blood rise rapidly. Indeed, this rapid rise gives an addictive hit – the faster the better! A video of blood sugar levels would look like the Rocky Mountains. Beer is particularly high in sugar and alcohol, and drunk quickly gives the best addictive hit of all carbohydrates. Many foods achieve the same hit and we call this 'comfort eating' – we use it to deal with stress.

Sugar, fruit sugar and refined carbohydrates (white flours, white rice, cooked potato and other root vegetables) are addictive – but especially sugar.

Whilst the brain loves this carbohydrate hit, it is highly damaging to the body. Insulin is poured out to deal with the sugar high. Importantly, the rate at which the blood sugar rises determines the amount of insulin released. Blood sugars come crashing down as insulin shunts sugar into fat cells via triglycerides (see page 206). The body is saved from sugar damage! But as blood sugar levels fall quickly, the brain goes into panic mode – it cannot afford to run out of energy as this means becoming unconscious and easy prey for the local sabre-toothed tiger. The main panic hormone is adrenaline (though there are many others).

We associate the falling blood sugars with adrenaline, and indeed adrenaline and other stress hormones are responsible for the symptoms we call hypoglycaemia.

Ultimately, these fluctuating levels of sugar, insulin, adrenaline and other stress hormones lead to metabolic syndrome, or 'syndrome X' – a clinical picture (see page 228) which is the major forerunner of disability and death in Western societies. Metabolic syndrome progresses to hypertension (high blood pressure), diabetes, obesity, cardiovascular disease, mental disorders, degenerative conditions (including arthritis and osteoporosis) and cancer. Alzheimer's disease has been dubbed 'type III diabetes'.

The symptoms of hypoglycaemia are varied and derive from the various mechanisms that give rise to the stress response and result from it.

SYMPTOMS OF HYPOGLYCAEMIA

- From adrenalin release: disturbed sleep, shakiness, anxiety, nervousness, palpitations, tachycardia, sweating, feeling of warmth, pallor, coldness, clamminess, dilated pupils, numb feelings, 'pins and needles'.
- From glucagon (see page 202) and other gut hormone release: hunger, rumbling gut, nausea, vomiting, abdominal discomfort, headache.
- From poor energy delivery to the body: as listed on page 2.
- From reduced energy delivery to the brain: as listed on page 46.

The upper fermenting gut (see page 201) makes all the above problems much worse because the alcohols produced by this inappropriate fermentation further destabilise blood sugar levels.

We can test for hypoglycaemia, but the clinical picture is usually very clear (see page 206).

TESTS FOR HYPOGLYCAEMIA

- A blood glucose level measured when symptoms occur may be misleading – it is the rate at which blood sugar levels fall that determines the amount of adrenaline released.
- Six-hour glucose tolerance test – a video is better than a snap shot. The future of diagnosis will lie with continuous blood sugar monitoring.
- Short-chain fatty acids (SCFAs)– measured in morning before breakfast. Where there is nocturnal hypoglycaemia, the body switches to SCFAs as a fuel, so levels of such may be low.

However, the clinical picture is so characteristic that I rarely request these tests. In particular, longstanding hypoglycaemia results in the clinical picture of metabolic syndrome, including:

- High body mass index (BMI), and being apple shaped – that is, fat is dumped where the immune system is busy; being apple shaped also points to upper fermenting gut.
- High LDL ('bad') cholesterol and low HDL ('good') cholesterol.
- Blood sugar levels that fluctuate rapidly.
- Variable blood pressure initially (the adrenalin released spikes blood sugar), then continuous high blood pressure as arteries become stiffened through scarring.
- High normal erythrocyte sedimentation rate (ESR – see page 48), high normal blood plasma viscosity – the 'normal range' for ESR has changed over time. It used to be 1–10 mm per hour. That has been increased to 1–20 mm per hour, rising with age. This reflects the fact that metabolic syndrome is now considered normal.
- Raised glycosylated haemoglobin.
- Levels of insulin inappropriate to blood sugar levels (insulin resistance).

The Paleo-ketogenic diet starts to address the problems resulting from allergy (because it is low allergen), hypoglycaemia and the upper fermenting gut (because it is low carb).

Having discussed the Paleo-ketogenic diet and hypoglycaemia, I will now look at the next aspect of 'fuel in the tank' – micronutrients.

Micronutrients

Westerners all need micronutrient supplements in addition to a Paleo-ketogenic diet because:

- Modern agriculture results in micronutrient-deficient crops.
- Food storage and processing further deplete micronutrient levels.
- We are physically inactive, we need less food and therefore consume fewer micronutrients.
- We are all inevitably exposed to more toxins in the environment, which require additional micronutrients to help detoxify them. These may be persistent organic pollutants (POPs – pesticides, volatile organic compounds, heavy metals), noxious gases, food additives, social addictions or prescribed medications. Many of these substances require micronutrients for their elimination from the body.

Micronutrient status can be determined through blood, sweat or urine testing. It is important to consult with the lab where the tests are done because some tests can be misleading. For example, a serum magnesium reading is unhelpful since serum magnesium is maintained at the expense of levels inside cells. Hair tests also can be misleading.

In addition to the above, there are some interesting evolutionary wrinkles which have implications for modern diets and routine supplements.

Vitamin C – During evolution, humans, together with fruit bats and guinea pigs, lost their ability to manufacture their own vitamin C. This explains why your dog does not get scurvy from eating a pure meat diet. Humans must now eat vegetables and berries to obtain vitamin C. I recommend a large single dose of vitamin C (2–6 grams, to bowel tolerance) at night to help maintain an upper gut that does not ferment. I suspect upper fermenting gut is the major risk factor for oesophageal, stomach and bowel cancer, the second commonest cancers in men and women.

Vitamin D – Humans evolved in Africa running naked under the African sunshine and developing a dark skin to protect themselves from burning in ultraviolet (UV) light. We evolved the ability to make vitamin D from the effect of UV light on cholesterol in the skin – vitamin D is markedly anti-inflammatory and further protected the skin from damaging inflammation in response to this UV. Vitamin D diffuses through the rest of the body, where it acts as a general anti-inflammatory. What this means clinically is that the further away from the Equator one lives, the greater the tendency to pro-inflammatory conditions. Sunshine is by far and away the most important source of vitamin D. One hour of Mediterranean sun produces about 10,000 IU (International Units) of vitamin D. As primitive man migrated away from the Equator he started to run into problems with vitamin D deficiency and a lighter skin evolved – so modern Mediterraneans are olivaceous, and Northeners white. Indeed, Northerners followed sea routes with high-fish diets so much of their vitamin D was fish derived. Most modern Caucasians are vitamin D deficient. There is an inverse relation between sunshine exposure, vitamin D levels, and incidence of disease as one moves away from the Equator. Vitamin D protects against osteoarthritis, osteoporosis, fractures (vitamin D improves muscle strength, thereby improving balance and movement and preventing falls), cancer, hypertension, high cholesterol, diabetes, heart disease, multiple sclerosis and susceptibility to infections. In the absence of sunshine, I recommend at least 2,000–10,000 IU of D3 daily.

Vitamin B3 is not, strictly speaking, a vitamin (a vital substance that we have
to consume because our bodies cannot make it). The body can synthesise
vitamin B3 (niacin, niacinamide) from the amino acid tryptophan. However,
it needs large amounts of protein to do so. Paleo-ketogenic diets were high
in protein; modern diets are lacking, and so now for most people niacin has
become a vitamin. I recommend 500 mg daily.

Glutathione is almost invariably deficient because it is in such demand to detoxify persistent organic pollutants (POPs). I recommend at least 250 mg daily.

Having covered micronutrient status, we come to the last sub-section of
'fuel in the tank' – namely, gut function. Here I shall deal with the problems
of the upper fermenting gut and hypochlorrhydria (stomach acid deficiency).

Gut function

THE UPPER FERMENTING GUT

Gastroenterologists like to call this 'small bowel bacterial overgrowth', but I
do not like that name because it excludes the possibility of fermentation in the
stomach and fermentation by yeast. The bacterium *Helicobacter pylori* is one
example of a fermenting microbe. However, I suspect yeast is the commonest
upper gut fermenting microbe. We can all develop a fermenting upper gut
if we eat sufficient carbohydrate to overwhelm the body's ability to digest
and absorb it. I do that when I eat too much at Christmas! However, lack of
stomach acid and pancreatic enzymes and bile salts, all of which kill microbes,
further predispose us to upper fermenting gut. So does poor energy delivery
since the business of digesting, absorbing and dealing with the results of such
in the liver is greatly demanding of energy. I suspect, with age, most people
eating Western diets develop upper fermenting gut.

The symptoms of the condition are:

- **Any gut symptom,** but particularly bloating as gases may be produced.
- **Fatigue** – Products of fermentation include various alcohols, hydrogen
  sulphide, D-lactate and other such which have the potential to inhibit
  mitochondria (see page 32).
- **Foggy brain** – The fermenting gut is also known as the 'auto-
  brewery syndrome'.
- **Hypoglycaemia** – Even when a good low glycaemic index diet is
  being followed.
- **Allergies** – We can become sensitised to gut microbes. I suspect this
  explains many allergic symptoms which do not respond to elimination
  diets, such as arthritis, polymyalgia rheumatica, interstitial cystitis, vulvitis,

prostatitis, connective tissue disease, temporal arteritis, urticaria, and possibly asthma, varicose eczema, acne and rosacea, tinnitus, age-related deafness and many others.

- **Susceptibility to infections** – Because ingested and inhaled microbes (which are coughed up and swallowed) that are not killed in a bath of stomach acid, bacteria can survive in the upper gut, causing fermentation. Many of my patients' CFS has been triggered by a gut virus, such as Epstein Barr (glandular fever).
- **Psychological and psychiatric disorders** – Work by the Japanese researcher Professor Nishihara[6] suggests that gut microbes appear in the brain with the potential to ferment brain neurotransmitters to neuro-active and psycho-active substances like LSD and amphetamine. This may explain a loss of touch with reality, such as severe mood swings, paranoia, hallucinations, obsessive compulsive disorders, eating disorders and behaviour disorders.

Tests for upper fermenting gut in order of clinical usefulness are:
- Comprehensive digestive stool analysis, which screens out major pathology, gives a good handle on ability to digest and absorb. It indicates which microbes are present, which are likely to be fermenting and their anti-microbial sensitivities (herbal and prescription)
- Breath tests for *H. pylori* and other upper gut fermenters
- Blood alcohol levels following a glucose load – Broadly speaking, yeasts ferment to ethanol; bacteria ferment to higher alcohols, such as various propanols and butanols
- Hydrogen breath test
- Hydrogen sulphide in the urine
- Measure D-lactate in the blood

However, no test is perfect, and we need more.

HYPOCHLORHYDRIA

We need an acid stomach for protein digestion, absorption of micronutrients and sterilising food to prevent infection. Insufficient acid – namely, hypochlorhydria – results in poor protein digestion, malabsorption of minerals and upper fermenting gut. Symptoms of acidity and acid reflux (GERD) may be due to what I call a 'half acid stomach'.

The normal oesophagus is neutral at pH 7. Normal stomach contents are extremely acid at pH 2–4; the normal duodenum is alkaline at pH 8. As foods are eaten and enter the stomach, the effect of the food arriving dilutes stomach contents and the pH rises. The stomach pours in acid to allow digestion of proteins to take place and the pH falls back down to its normal value of 2–4. The key to understanding GERD is the pyloric sphincter, which is the muscle which controls emptying of the stomach into the duodenum. This muscle is acid-sensitive and it only relaxes when the acidity of the stomach is correct – that is, pH 2–4. At this point stomach contents can empty into the duodenum (where they are neutralised by bicarbonate released from the liver via bile ducts).

If the stomach does not produce enough acid and the pH is only, say 5, then the muscle which allows the stomach to empty (the pyloric sphincter) will not open. When the stomach contracts in order to move food into the duodenum, the progress of the food will be blocked by this contracted pyloric sphincter. But of course, the pressure in the stomach increases and the food gets squirted back up into the oesophagus. Although this food is not very acid (not acid enough to relax the pyloric sphincter), it is sufficiently acid to burn the oesophagus and so one gets the symptoms of gastro-oesophageal reflux. The paradox is that this symptom is caused by not enough stomach acid – that is, the reverse of what is generally believed.

Acid blockers, such as proton-pump inhibitors and H2 blockers, may afford short-term relief from hyper-acidity symptoms but spell disaster for gut function. Minerals are malabsorbed (resulting in osteoporosis), proteins are not broken down (resulting in allergies as large antigenically interesting molecules appear downstream) and the gut is not sterilised, resulting in fermenting gut and susceptibility to infection.

In the duodenum and small intestine, pancreatic enzymes and bile salts are essential to emulsify, digest and absorb fats, essential fatty acids and fat-soluble vitamins. They further help reduce numbers of microbes in the upper gut.

We can test for hypochlorhydia as follows:

- Swallowing bicarbonate, say half a teaspoon in half a pint of water, on a fasting, empty stomach, should result in belching within two minutes as carbon dioxide is released by the action of acid on bicarbonate
- Measuring salivary VEGF (a saliva sample)
- Finding meat fibres present in a stool analysis (but this may also be due to poor pancreatic function)
- Using a pH string test

So, depending on these test results, it may be necessary to test for pancreatic function as follows:

- Faecal elastase.
- Comprehensive digestive stool analysis – To measure levels of enzymes and bile salts, together with the presence of meat fibres and fats.
- Amylase – This is a test of damage to the pancreas and is only abnormal where there is severe pathology.

2. Regular servicing of our engines – sleep

Sleep is the golden chain that ties health and our bodies together.

THOMAS DEKKER (1572–1632)

All living creatures have times in their cycle when they shut down their metabolic activity for healing and repair to take place. In higher animals we call this sleep. During the 'flu epidemic after the First World War, a few sufferers developed neurological damage in which they lost the ability to sleep. All were dead within two weeks. This was the first solid evidence that sleep is an absolute essential for life. Happily the body has a symptom which tells us how much sleep we need. It is called tiredness – ignore this at your peril! During sleep we heal and repair; during our waking hours we cause cell damage. If there is insufficient sleep, then the cell damage exceeds healing and repair and our health gradually ratchets downhill. Lack of sleep is a major risk factor for all degenerative conditions, from heart disease to cancer to neurological disorders.

Without a good night's sleep on a regular basis all other interventions are to no avail.

Humans evolved to sleep when it is dark and wake when it is light. Sleep is a form of hibernation, when the body shuts down in order to repair damage done through use, to conserve energy and to hide from predators. The normal sleep pattern that evolved in hot climates is to sleep, keep warm and conserve energy during the cold nights and then sleep again in the afternoons when it is too hot to work and to hide away from the midday sun. As humans migrated away from the Equator, the sleep pattern had to change with the seasons and as the lengths of the days changed. In winter we need to shut down to conserve energy – this means more sleep. Mild fatigue and depression prevent us from spending energy unnecessarily. Conversely, in the summer we need to expend large amounts of energy to harvest the summer bounties and accumulate reserves to carry us through the winter; we naturally need less sleep, can work longer hours and have more energy. But the need for a rest (if not a sleep) in the middle of the day is still there. Therefore it is no surprise that young children, the elderly and people who are ill often have an extra sleep in the afternoon, and for these people that is totally desirable. Others have learned to 'power nap', as it is called, during the day, and this allows them to feel more energetic later. If you can do it then this is an excellent habit to get into – and it can be learned. The average daily sleep requirement is nine hours, ideally taken between 9.30 pm and 6.30 am – that is, during the hours of darkness – but allow for more in the winter and less in the summer. An hour of sleep before midnight is worth two after – this is because human growth hormone is produced during the hours of sleep before midnight.

To show how important the balance of hours of sleep and rest are, divide the day into 12 hours of activity and 12 hours of rest. If you have one extra hour of activity (13 hours), you lose an hour of rest and sleep (11 hours). The difference is two hours!

There are two very easy ways to spot symptoms of insufficient sleep:

- reliance on an alarm clock to wake in the morning
- looking forward to sleeping in on non-work days

3. The engine of our car – mitochondria

All mammals are made up of about 300 different cell types – muscle cells, nerve cells, skin cells and so on – all of which have a different job of work to do. Whatever that job happens to be, it will require energy. The way that energy is supplied to cells is the same for all cells and, indeed, for all living creatures. Energy is delivered by tiny engines within cells that take fuel from the blood stream and burn it in the presence of oxygen to make energy in the form of a substance called adenotriphosphate or ATP. These engines are called mitochondria. The mitochondria in my editor and ABBA-fan Craig's pet frog, Frida, are the same as those in me. A heart cell may contain 2,000 to 3,000 mitochondria and a heart by weight is 25 per cent mitochondria.

ATP is the currency of energy in the body. With ATP we can buy any job, from contracting a muscle to making a hormone. ATP is present in every living cell and makes the difference between a living cell and a dead one. Indeed, if ATP levels fall low this triggers apoptosis – that is, cell suicide. If energy delivery is impaired, then the cell will go slow; if the cell goes slow, then the organ goes slow. Poor ATP delivery – that is, poor energy delivery – can therefore result in many different symptoms.

For good energy delivery, not only must the mitochondria be working well, but there must be enough of them. The business of getting physically and mentally fit and staying fit is all about putting in place interventions to allow mitochondria to work to their full potential, and then getting more of them.

CFS patients are not hypochondriacs but mitochondriacs!

I have learned so much about mitochondria from two books. Firstly, consultant cardiologist Dr Stephen Sinatra in his book *The Sinatra Solution*. Then from Professor Nick Lane's book *Power, Sex, Suicide*, which further elucidates the wonderful biochemistry and evolutionary imperatives that resulted in our magnificent mitochondrial machines.

Why mitochondria go slow and how to test for this

In 2009, Dr John McLaren-Howard, Dr Norman Booth and I published a paper about mitochondrial function in CFS patients: www.ncbi.nlm.nih .gov/pmc/articles/PMC2680051. We published again in 2012: www.ijcem .com/files/IJCEM1204005.pdf. What these papers showed is that those CFS patients with the worst levels of energy had the worst mitochondrial function, and vice versa. It was the first paper to be published with objective measureable evidence of poor energy delivery at the cellular level and how this translated into the clinical symptom of fatigue. Our third paper demonstrated that those people undertaking the necessary interventions to address mitochondrial function improved biochemically and clinically: www.ijcem .com/files/IJCEM1207003.pdf.

This paper was possible because of the brilliance of Dr John McLaren-Howard, who developed a test – namely, **'ATP profiles'** – which is able to measure how well mitochondria work. It is not good enough to measure absolute levels of ATP in cells since this will simply reflect immediate ATP available and therefore only how well rested the sufferer is.

John measures: how efficiently ATP is made within mitochondria; how well ATP is transported out of mitochondria and across the mitochondrial membrane into the cell where it is used; how well energy can be released from ATP (a magnesium-dependent process within the cell) when transformed into ADP (adenodiphosphate); and how well ADP is transported back across the mitochondrial membrane into mitochondria. Mitochondrial membranes are 80 per cent composed of translocator proteins that do nothing but shunt ATP and ADP to and fro from where it is produced to where it is needed and back again.

By measuring these various parameters and scoring them, it is possible objectively to assess how much energy is available to cells. Some of my severe CFS patients have as little as 10 per cent of available energy compared with the lowest limit of the population range – it is no wonder they are wiped out.

Mitochondria can go slow for a number of reasons. John has developed further tests to explore these reasons:

Not enough raw materials for mitochondria to work – The common rate-limiting issues are deficiencies of magnesium, vitamin B3, acetyl-L-carnitine, coenzyme Q10 and D-ribose. However, there will be others.

> *Tests*: Measure the above. The need for D-ribose is inferred from levels of ATP.

The mitochondria are blocked by a toxin – Such toxins can come from the body (for example, aldehydes from poor antioxidant status or products of the upper fermenting gut) or from outside the body (such as pesticides, heavy metals or volatile organic substances). Mitochondria can also be blocked by lactic acid. This represents just one of the many vicious cycles we see in CFS patients – the more one slips into anaerobic metabolism the harder it is to get out of it.

> *Tests*: Translocator protein studies, or microrespirometry studies.

Mitochondrial membranes are the wrong shape – It is membranes that hold the bundles of enzymes (cristae) in just the right 3D configuration to allow all the biochemical steps to proceed efficiently. These membranes contain cardiolipin, a substance that is unique to mitochondria. The right combination of fats is needed to achieve this. Cardiolipin studies shed light on mitochondrial membrane structure.

> *Test*: Cardiolipin studies

How to increase the number of mitochondria

The body is extraordinarily efficient. It cannot afford any metabolic waste – this is so that energy and reserves can be preserved for the lean times ahead. This ploy has been essential in evolutionary terms to allow survival. However, we now live in a time of plenty and we can afford to be mentally and physically lazy. Modern humans have to be disciplined to use their brains and bodies or they will cease to function at full potential. If you don't use it, you lose it.

What is interesting is the amount one has to do to remain physically fit – remarkably little. What stimulates the production of more mitochondria is lactic acid. This approach makes perfect evolutionary sense. I do not see badgers and foxes trotting round my hill and doing press-ups every morning to get fit. Most of the time wild animals are in hiding or feeding quietly. Around once a week there will be a predator-prey interaction – the predator must run for his life to get his breakfast; the prey must run for his life to avoid being breakfast! In doing so, both parties will achieve maximal lactic acid burn. This is all that is required to get fit and stay fit. It is possible to get physically fit in 12 minutes a week with the right sort of exercise.

Low numbers of mitochondria may be a symptom of hypothyroidism, which will require further investigation and treatment.

Energy delivery to the brain – the importance of fats

There is a further interesting peculiarity with respect to the energy supply to the brain, which is different from that used by the rest of the body. As I have said already, although the brain weighs just 2 per cent of total body weight, it uses 20 per cent of the total energy generated in the body. There are not enough mitochondria in the brain to explain this, which means there must be another energy-generating source. Brain cells are also very different from normal cells. They have a cell body, and a very long tail – or dendrite – which communicate with other cells. Indeed, if a nerve-cell body from my spinal cord that supplied my toes was sitting on my desk in England and was the size of a football, the tail would be in New York! These tails (dendrites) are too narrow to contain mitochondria, but it has been suggested that the energy supply comes directly from the myelin (fatty) sheaths which wrap around nerve fibres. Myelin has adopted mitochondrial biochemistry to produce ATP and it is this that supplies the energy for neuro-transmission. Myelin sheaths are made up almost entirely of fats, so we need to look to oils and fats for improved energy supply to brain cells.

As far as we know, humans evolved on the East Coast of Africa, eating a diet rich in sea food. It is suggested that the high levels of oils, particularly fish oils, allowed the brain to develop fast. Primitive humans came to have bigger brains so allowing intelligence to develop. Essential fatty acids are vital for normal brain function. We need two types of fat for good brain function – firstly, medium-chain fats as fuels, such as meat fat (lard and dripping), butter, coconut oil, palm oil and chocolate fat; and secondly, fats for building membranes for energy delivery in the myelin sheaths – these are long-chain fats found in vegetables, fish, nut and seed oils.

Our modern phobia of cholesterol and fat is producing an epidemic of depression and dementia.

To see if there are deficiencies or imbalances in essential fatty acids it is necessary to measure blood levels of erythrocyte (red blood cell) and essential fatty acid levels.

4. Oxygen supply and fuel delivery
– heart, lungs, blood and blood vessels

Oxygen – even I know what happens when my cylinder runs out.

Patient (former miner) with pneumoconiosis c. 1985

Oxygen and fuel delivery require a healthy pair of lungs for oxygen exchange to take place, good oxygen-carrying capacity – that is, good levels of haemo-globin in the blood – open arteries and a strongly pumping heart. Symptoms of failures of the above would include all the symptoms of poor energy delivery. In addition, one may see pallor or cold extremities, and in extreme cases blueness, or 'cyanosis', of extremities and lips. Problems that can arise include:

Heart – This is one area where there is an obvious vicious cycle for my CFS patients – poor energy delivery to the heart means that it does not beat strongly as a pump and therefore this will further impair fuel and oxygen delivery and therefore worsen mitochondrial function. This explains the symptoms of 'postural orthostatic tachycardia syndrome' often seen in severe CFS. The heart cannot increase output by beating more strongly because it does not have the energy delivery to do so. It tries to increase output by beating more quickly, but this is only sustainable for a few minutes or seconds. Blood pressure then drops precipitously and the patient has to lie down or he/she will black out.

Lungs – The lungs are designed for peak athletic performance. In Nature we achieve this roughly once a week where there is a predator–prey interaction – you have to literally run for your life, either to save it or to secure your next meal. What this means is that at rest the lungs only have to achieve a fraction of what is needed during fight or flight. Unfortunately, this means that a great deal of lung damage can be sustained before that person realises what is going on (especially if they do not exercise to test the system). So, for example, chronic obstructive pulmonary disease (COPD) and emphysema often first present after years of smoking damage to the lungs. Poor lung function is usually an obvious cause of poor energy delivery.

Blood vessels – The main cause of impaired blood supply to the organs in Westerners is hardening of the arteries, or atherosclerosis. Arteries have a delicate lining which can be easily damaged by turbulent blood flow. Of course, this is going to happen when the blood pressure increases and typically occurs where one blood vessel divides into two and therefore there is more turbulence at this junction. High blood pressure can occur as a result of stress because the stress hormone adrenaline is released. The commonest cause of adrenaline release is fluctuating blood sugar levels with hypoglycaemia. (There's another double whammy here – if blood sugar levels spike then this will damage the artery directly – it is sticky stuff and forms AGEs [advanced glycation end products – see page 191].) So, with high-carbohydrate diets the arteries are damaged by the sugar and then again by the turbulent flow created by high blood pressure. Pathology arises when the immune system moves in to heal these areas of damage – the healing and repair process involves laying down fibrous tissue and this will narrow the blood vessel slightly, leading to more turbulence and more damage. This is why controlling blood pressure and blood sugar are such an important part of preventing arterial damage. The combination of high blood pressure, loss of control of blood sugars and obesity we call **metabolic syndrome**, which results in a host of other problems subsequently.

Anaemia – Insufficient haemoglobin (the oxygen-carrying molecule) may arise because of insufficient raw material (iron or vitamin B12), low numbers of red cells (poor bone marrow function) or abnormal haemoglobin (sickle cell anaemia, thalassaemia) or haemolytic anaemia (several possible causes).

Hyperventilation – If we over-breathe, carbon dioxide is washed out of our blood stream. This makes the blood more alkaline and in turn makes oxygen stick more avidly to haemoglobin, so it is not available to cells. Hyperventilation is a stress response which in Nature would occur most often in preparation for flight or fight. The lactic acid produced by such would mitigate the alkalosis of hyperventilation.

TESTS FOR PROBLEMS WITH OXYGEN SUPPLY AND FUEL DELIVERY

Investigations include:

- **For anaemia** – full blood count. Anaemia is a symptom that must always be taken seriously because unrecognised blood loss may be the first symptom of serious pathology. This always needs investigating as a matter of urgency.
- **Nutritional causes of anaemia** – measure ferritin and serum B12.
- Consider **poor energy delivery to the bone marrow** – Bone marrow is greatly demanding of energy to make new blood. I suspect this explains the anaemia of chronic disease.
- **Arterial function** – Doppler scans for blood flow, angiograms.
- **Heart function** – The best test for whether the heart is pumping strongly is exercise. Inability to get fit, or inability to walk briskly up a hill without serious shortness of breath or pain, could point to poor cardiac reserve.
- **Lung function tests** – The best test of lung function is again exercise tolerance. 'Pink puffers' represent the smokers' disease of emphysema

(heart OK); 'blue bloaters' have poor cardiac output (lungs OK).
Lung function tests available through a respiratory physiologist are
very helpful.
• **Red cell carbonic anhydrase studies** can help to diagnose hyperventilation.

5. The accelerator pedal of our car – the thyroid gland

Engines work most efficiently when they go at their optimal speed. In the
body, the thyroid gland controls the rate of metabolism so both an underactive
and an overactive thyroid are major risk factors for disease. Both conditions
impact hugely on energy delivery. The problems of underactive thyroid are
much more common than overactive.

Diagnosing a thyroid problem is not straightforward. The biggest mistake
that doctors make is to rely exclusively on blood tests. The clinical picture is
just as important, and for some patients one can only know by prescribing a
trial of thyroid hormones.

Reasons for the current thyroid disease epidemic

We are seeing an epidemic of thyroid disease likely because of:

Micronutrient deficiency – Iodine is essential for thyroid function and iodine
deficiency is almost pandemic. Other micronutrients are also important,
especially zinc, iron and selenium.

   Test: Iodine in urine, plasma zinc, ferritin, red cell selenium.

Toxic stress – The normal function of thyroid hormones depends on: a normal hypothalamic-pituitary-adrenal axis for control; normal thyroid gland
for production; and normal transport and receptor function for hormones
to have an effect. These actions can be variously blocked by other halides
(chemicals in the same family as iodine) such as fluoride (drinking water,
toothpaste and dental treatments), bromide (PBBs), radioactive iodine
(medical treatments, Chernobyl, Fukoshima). Other chemical thyroid
insults include perchlorates (washing powder and rocket fuel), phthalates
and bisphenol A (in plastic wrappings), pyridines (cigarette smoke), PCBs
and PBBs (fire retardants in soft furnishing), UV screens (sunblocks), cosmetics, pesticides and probably many more.

   Test: Toxic metals in urine following DMSA (see page 197); fat biopsy
        for pesticides and VOCs (volatile organic compounds).

Autoimmune hypothyroidism – This too is becoming increasingly common. It
should be treated as for the general approach to autoimmunity: Paleo-ketogenic

diet; avoid adjuvants as in immunisations and silicones; detox pesticides and toxic metals; improve antioxidant status; and high-dose vitamin D.

Test: Autoantibody screen.

Viral thyroiditis – The increasing world population and more travel means more novel viruses.

Thyroid hormone receptor resistance – The idea here is similar to the problem of type II diabetes, in which insulin levels are normal but the receptor is blocked; this is called 'insulin resistance'. This may result from any of the chemical insults listed above. There is no test to measure it; at present diagnosis relies on a trial of pure T3 thyroid hormone.

Natural goitrogens – Soya products are a key example (fermented soya may be less of a problem).

Signs and symptoms of underactive thyroid

The signs and symptoms of an underactive thyroid result from poor energy delivery (see page 2).

There are some additional symptoms which are typical of an underactive thyroid: weight gain; fluid retention (myxoedema); loss of eyebrows; thin, dry hair; dry skin; headaches; vertigo and deafness; constipation; menstrual problems and premenstrual tension (PMT); infertility and loss of libido.

Signs of an underactive thyroid include: puffy face or puffy eyes; dry skin; rashes, eczema and boils; enlargement of the tongue ('macroglossia' – if the patient sticks her tongue out, it will fill her mouth and touch the lip corners); hoarse voice, voice change, loss of singing voice; slow heart rate; goitre (swelling at the base of the neck); slowed Achilles tendon reflex; low basal body temperature; and almost anything else!

Tests of thyroid function

A blood test to measure thyroid hormone levels – namely, free T4, free T3 and TSH (thyroid-stimulating hormone) – is an essential start. However, for the purposes of treatment the clinical detail is as important, arguably more important, as the blood tests.

6. The gear box of the car – the adrenal glands

The body has to work efficiently and gear energy delivery to energy demand. By doing so, reserves are conserved for lean times and this has been vital to evolutionary success. In moments of acute stress, such as being chased by a sabre-toothed tiger, we need to maximise energy delivery.

To achieve peak performance there is an outpouring of the instant stress hormone, adrenaline. If the hunt continues there is an outpouring of the medium-term stress hormone hydrocortisone. If the stress continues further then there is an outpouring of the long-term stress hormone DHEA (dehydroepiandrosterone).

Such an outpouring of hormones allows mitochondria to increase their output by 200 per cent. This explains why it is generally only at world events that world records are broken.

However, this is not sustainable in the long term. Unremitting stress results in adrenal exhaustion – indeed, this may be a way of protecting mitochondria; if ATP levels fall too low then cells will die.

A normally functioning adrenal gland is essential for life. No function (as in Addison's disease) kills; too much (as in Cushing's syndrome or with taking steroid hormones) maims. What I see most commonly is adrenal exhaustion – that is, partial failure, resulting from chronic unremitting stress.

A certain amount of stress is essential for healthy and productive life. Getting the balance right is the tricky bit. Stress can come in many guises. Essentially the symptom of stress arises when energy demand exceeds, or potentially exceeds, energy delivery.

The main stressors, in order of clinical frequency, are:

- Fluctuating blood sugar levels – because of sugar and carbohydrate addiction, resulting in lack of sleep – either poor quality or insufficient hours of sleep or both.
- Other addictions – alcohol, nicotine, drugs, prescription medications. Ironically, we use all these to cope with the symptoms of stress because they allow our brains to ignore those distressing symptoms, but this creates further obvious vicious cycles.
- Emotional and psychological stress.
- Financial and time stress.
- Infectious stress – often it is the viral infection which is the last straw that breaks the camel's back and tips an under-functioning person into a full blown CFS patient. Rarely is the virus the sole cause.
- Micronutrient deficiencies.
- Undiagnosed allergies.
- Toxic stress and poisoning – from environmental exposures (polluting industry), occupational exposures (pesticides), social exposures (cosmetics, hair dyes), and prescription medications.
- And there are many other possibilities!

Symptoms of adrenal fatigue

Symptoms of adrenal fatigue (partial failure of the adrenal glands) include:
- All the symptoms of poor energy delivery (see page 2).
- In addition – inability to rise to the challenge and deal with any of the above stressors.
- Loss of the ability to get excited – this is the symptom related to adrenaline deficiency.
- I suspect poor temperature control, with a tendency to excessive sweating.

Coping with stress

We use addictions to cope with stress. Addictions stop us caring. They give us immediate relief – a smoker will tell you that the comfortable sensation starts within milliseconds of inhalation and, indeed, even in anticipation of relief. Addictions mask the very symptoms which tell us something is going wrong and lead us into further disease. However, the relief does not last and a further dose of addiction is necessary to feel 'normal'.

We all know this, but it does not prevent addiction. The power of short-term emotional gain is much stronger than cold-blooded intellectual knowledge. It takes an iron will and much self-discipline to start to deal with addictions.

Many prescription drugs are addictive and simply replace one addiction with another.

I see the Western progression though life as an addictive ladder which starts with sugar and refined carbohydrates and moves up through nicotine, alcohol, cannabis, ecstasy and heroin. The addict either dies prematurely or realises his errors and climbs back down the addiction ladder, but often is left on the first rung of sugar and refined carbohydrate. In terms of scale this is the most serious addiction because it is not recognised as such – indeed, it is socially acceptable.

The good news is that adrenaline is also an addiction. One strategy is to swap unhealthy for healthy addictions, like exercise, pets, the Arts and Culture. These healthy addictions are even better if there is a competitive edge. I go team chasing on my horse.

TESTS FOR POOR ADRENAL FUNCTION

Conventional testing for adrenal function relies on a short synacthen test in which the patient is injected with ACTH, a hormone that gives the adrenal gland a powerful kick. This will pick up complete adrenal failure, as occurs in Addison's disease, but will not pick up partial failure or adrenal fatigue. A useful test, which is easily done on a saliva sample, is an 'adrenal stress profile', which measures levels of cortisol and DHEA over 24 hours. One expects to see highest levels in the morning, which taper through the day. Too high a result of either indicates a stress response; too little indicates adrenal fatigue.

Treatment is about identifying and dealing with the cause of the stress upstream. In the short term, physiological doses of cortisol or DHEA are often helpful. More recently I have started using pregnenolone – metabolically, this is immediately downstream of the raw material cholesterol from which all steroid hormones are synthesised.

It is T3 (activated thyroid hormone) which kicks the adrenal gland into life and spikes the levels of cortisol and DHEA to wake us up. Low morning levels of cortisol and DHEA may point to hypothyroidism.

7. The exhaust system: detoxing – liver and kidney function
Sources of toxic stress

The gut, I suspect, is the largest source of toxic stress. Blood draining from the gut passes in the portal vein directly to the liver to deal with such. At rest, the liver consumes a massive amount of energy – 29 per cent of total energy consumption – to deal with this toxic load.

If you look at life from the point of view of a plant, it does not want to be eaten and renders itself as poisonous as possible. Indeed, the vast majority of plant matter in the world is too toxic to eat. Even foods that we do eat regularly contain toxins, such as lectins, alkaloids and possible carcinogens. As I mentioned before, the cycad seed consumed on the island of Guam causes motor neurone disease.

Toxic stress also results from the fermenting gut. We normally ferment vegetable fibre in the lower gut to produce fuel in the form of short-chain fatty acids – one such, n-butyrate, is essential for nourishing the lining of the large bowel. However, where there is abnormal fermentation in the upper gut (stomach and small intestine) of carbohydrates and proteins, there is production of many toxins such as ethyl, propyl and butyl alcohols, hydrogen sulphide, D-lactate, oxalates and many others.

Normal metabolism of protein and carbohydrates – together with breakdown products of hormones, neurotransmitters, enzymes, haemoglobin and muscle fibres – results in many breakdown products, all of which have to be detoxified, recycled or excreted. These include urea, creatinine, uric acid, oxalates, purines and porphyrins, together with alcohols, esters and many others.

The above functions are carried out largely by the liver and kidneys. Both organs are greatly demanding of energy. We also know that liver is an extremely nourishing food because it is rich in all vitamins, minerals and essential fatty acids to allow it to function. All machines require a plentiful supply of energy and raw materials. The kidneys too are greatly demanding of energy; it is essential that they have a constant supply. They do not tolerate anything less. So, for example, a patient who develops acute low blood pressure will often damage his kidneys irreparably and go into kidney failure.

The gut too requires energy to function – indeed, in its ability to absorb essential nutrients and reject the rest the gut is like a giant nephron. (The kidneys are made up of hundreds of tiny nephrons – tubules that filter toxins from our blood.)

TESTS FOR LIVER AND KIDNEY FUNCTION (UREA, CREATININE, EGFR)

Uric acid; glutathione studies; detoxification profile to look at type one and type two detox ability; and other tests.

Gilbert's syndrome

Gilbert's syndrome may affect up to 10 per cent of the population. Although this is said to be a benign biochemical abnormality, actually it is symptomatic of an inability to detox through the process of 'glucuronidation' (the addition of glucoronic acid to a chemical to render it water soluble and therefore excreteable in urine). Sufferers are less able to clear a toxic load and so more susceptible to poisoning from endogenous (produced within the body) or exogenous (from outside the body) toxins. Most suffer from fatigue and it is common in my CFS patients.

TEST FOR GILBERT'S SYNDROME

Levels of bilirubin run high or high normal.

Mitochondria

Our detox systems evolved in response to toxins and waste products generated within the body. Any machine, to be running smoothly, requires not only a constant supply of materials but a tidying up of waste products. No machine is 100 per cent efficient, and the business of burning sugar in mitochondria in the presence of oxygen will produce toxins in the form of free radicals. These are mopped up by antioxidant systems within cells, extracellular fluid and the blood stream.

TESTS OF ANTIOXIDANT STATUS

The frontline antioxidants are superoxide dismutase, glutathione peroxidase and coenzyme Q10.

Cell damage

When cells are damaged or replaced through wear and tear, injury or inflammation, large molecules are released which are too big to get into the blood stream. These are mopped up by the lymphatic system – a system of drains which course throughout the body. The contents are broken down for recycling in lymph nodes to produce what is known as 'chyle', and finally empty into the inferior vena cava vein in the neck via the thoracic duct. Lymphatic drainage, as developed by Raymond Perrin PhD, is a massage technique to facilitate this natural flow.

TEST FOR CELL DAMAGE

The key symptom of this is cell-free DNA. My CFS patients often have high levels of cell-free DNA, comparable to that of patients on chemotherapy or following major physical trauma. It is very unusual to see a normal cell-free DNA in CFS. This test alone puts CFS in the category of major pathology.

Pollutants from the outside world

Because we live in an increasingly polluted world, we are putting more stress on our detox systems. These systems did not evolve to deal with such. However hard we try, we are all contaminated with pesticides, volatile organic compounds (VOCs) and heavy metals, which bio-accumulate in our tissues. I have yet to find a single person with a normal fat biopsy or absence of toxic metals in urine after taking a chelating agent (a substance that attracts and collects toxins and takes them with it out of the body). In addition, there are noxious gases.

As if this were not enough, we consume toxins such as food additives, alcohol, caffeine, prescription drugs and other such. It may be that in isolation these are not particularly toxic, but they have to be cleared by the body by the same mechanisms as more toxic substances. This creates a biochemical bottleneck – it takes longer for the total load to reduce, so toxins hang around longer with greater potential for harm.

As I said earlier, some toxins get into the body, do severe damage but evaporate or are detoxified before testing is possible. Such toxins include formaldehyde, noxious gases like carbon monoxide, sulphur dioxide and nitrous oxide, and radiation damage. Drugs of addiction, such as heroin, cannabis and ecstasy, have the potential for permanent damage (including death) but again may be undetectable by the time of testing.

There are no tests for silicone diffusing from implants. We know that anyone with silicone implants will have silicone widely distributed in the body. The question is whether it is triggering inflammation in the body. This we can test for by a silicone sensitivity test which measures the response of white cells to silicone.

TESTS OF EXOGENOUS TOXIC LOAD

A detailed, accurate patient history is a very good guide. It gives an idea of what exposures have taken place, with implications for avoidance and detox regimes. However, results of tests constantly surprise me. (The commonest source of *endogenous* toxins is the upper fermenting gut.)

TESTS FOR EXOGENOUS TOXINS

The clinically useful tests I regularly use to measure exogenous toxins are:

Fat biopsy for pesticides and VOCs: This is a very simple test to do – a 21G 0.8 mm green needle is pushed into buttock fat and removed. The amount of fat contained within the bore of the needle is sufficient for analysis. (Note, this test does not pick up heavy metals because they are not significantly present in fat.) Pesticides and VOCs are present in our fat in mg/kg. This would be similar to the sort of levels we would expect to see in blood if we were taking a therapeutic drug.

Toxic metals in urine after taking a chelating agent: Measuring toxic metals in urine, blood and hair is unreliable because heavy metals are very poorly excreted and bio-concentrate in organs such as heart, brain, bone marrow and kidney; they are therefore not available to measure. The answer is to use a chelating agent, such as DMSA, which is well absorbed from the gut, grabs toxic and friendly minerals alike, and pulls them out via the urine. It is excellent for diagnosing toxicity of heavy metals such as mercury, lead, arsenic, aluminium, cadmium, nickel and probably others.

DNA adducts: This is a measure of what is stuck onto DNA and may be blocking it doing its work. I do this test in any condition that may be associated with damage to DNA, such as cancer. Gene studies of superoxide dismutase often show evidence of gene blocking so DNA adducts is a logical follow-up test.

Translocator protein studies: These are indicated if mitochondrial function tests show blockage of TL protein. Using Raman spectroscopy and other techniques, Acumen Laboratories can identify a wide range of toxins, from oxidised lipids to toxic chemicals.

TESTS OF ABILITY TO DETOX

Standard blood tests of biochemistry (urea and electrolytes, liver function tests, kidney function tests, etc) give some handle on ability to detox:

Urea and creatinine levels: These are a measure of kidney function. Using an algorithm, glomerular filtration rate can be calculated from the creatinine level, age and sex. It should be above 90 ml/minute. In my severe CFS patients, I often see a low glomerular filtration rate. This makes good sense – if energy delivery is poor then the kidneys will go slow.

Bilirubin: In the absence of liver disease, a high bilirubin level indicates Gilbert's syndrome. Even a high-normal bilirubin level points to slow detox.

Gamma glutamyl transferase: This enzyme is induced in response to a toxic load – typically it is raised in response to excessive alcohol consumption. Some prescription medication has the same effect.

Glutathione S transferase: Levels may be high and this too may point to a toxic load.

Lactate dehydrogenase: This is the enzyme necessary to clear lactate, which results when there is a switch into anaerobic metabolism, with vast amounts of lactate produced. (Efficient energy production from glucose requires oxygen, and so is called 'aerobic'. Without sufficient oxygen it is 'anaerobic' and much less efficient.) I suspect high levels of this enzyme are symptomatic of such a tendency and point to poor mitochondrial function.

Glutathione: This needs to be in abundant supply but is commonly deficient.

Liver detoxification profile: This measures the ability of the body to excrete substances such as aspirin, caffeine and paracetamol so one can infer which enzyme pathways are deficient.

8. The driver of the car – the brain

What we think goes on in the world is not what actually goes on; it's what our brain tells us goes on. The best example of this is phantom limb syndrome, in which a limb has been lost but the brain tells the poor sufferer that it is still present. Sometimes it is perceived to be in an awkward position, or has an itch or a pain associated. This syndrome can be effectively treated by tricking the brain back into thinking normally, using mirrors. I think of this as remapping the brain.

Life experiences, particularly unpleasant ones, may remap the brain in such a way to result in unnecessary discomfort. For example, childhood trauma hardwires the brain for hyper-vigilance – this disturbs sleep and punches an emotional hole in our energy pot. Not surprisingly then, childhood trauma is a major risk factor for CFS. It is beyond the scope of this book to look at all the psychological therapies to rewire the brain to make life more comfortable, but they should not be forgotten in the treatment of any disease. However, what I see much more frequently in clinical practice is the opposite – obvious physical causes of disease are rejected in favour of a psychological explanation.

B. Mechanisms of energy expenditure

1. The immunological hole in the energy bucket

The immune system: our standing army – essential for defence but dangerous when aroused

The immune system is made up of intelligent, communicative, decision-making cells which, like the standing army of a country, may be activated to fight when needed. Like any army, the immune system is greatly demanding of energy and resources. Being so energy demanding, like the brain, it runs on fat, so fat is deposited where the immune system is active. (I suspect this explains the apple-shaped body we see in people with upper fermenting gut.) Ninety per cent of the immune system is associated with the gut. Bone marrow and lymph nodes, where immune cells are built and programmed, are buried in fat.

The jobs of the immune system

Healing and repair – The business of our making energy, detoxing molecules and physically moving around will damage tissues. The immune system is responsible for repair of such and this occurs during sleep.

Fighting off infection – The immune system is additionally employed when the frontline defences have been breached. This may be essential to fight off foreign pathogens but is also potentially dangerous to the body for two reasons. Firstly, too much inflammation causes tissue damage. Secondly, 'useless' inflammation may be switched on, such as allergy and auto-immunity. This is civil war – see below.

Allergy and autoimmunity – There has to be just the right amount of inflam-mation to kill off invaders effectively (so we don't end up with chronic infection), but not so much as to switch on allergy and autoimmunity. Many modern disease processes result from this lack of balance.

Immunological and biochemical fire – The NO/ON/OO pro-inflammatory cycle (page 220) – Professor Martin Pall brilliantly identified this biochem-ical pro-inflammatory cycle, which explains how some pro-inflammatory disease processes seem to have a momentum of their own. Even when the trigger has been identified and removed the inflammation continues. I think of this cycle as a biochemical fire which, once lit and fuelled, is difficult to put out. Western lifestyles are markedly pro-inflammatory. For the biochemists, the central players in the NO/ON/OO cycle are nitric oxide, peroxynitrite, superoxides and NF kappa B, which impact on pro-inflammatory receptors such as the vanilloid and NMDA receptors. They wind each other up!

Putting the fire out with antioxidants

What helps to keep our inflammatory cycles cool is our fire-fighting antioxidant system. Inflammation produces free radicals – these are highly damaging molecules. They are essential as the bullets that the immune system uses to shoot bacteria and viruses with. Free radicals are mopped up by antioxidants, but if these are lacking then there is potential for damage from friendly fire. Too much inflammation can be counter-productive. One example of too much inflammation in healing and repair is keloid scarring. In horses one sees proud flesh. Too much inflammation in response to infection may also kill by producing a cytokine storm – indeed, this is the mechanism that allowed the 1918 Spanish 'flu epidemic to kill 50–100 million people.

The frontline antioxidants which mop up free radicals are super-oxide dismutase (three types – within cells, within mitochondria, and outside cells), glutathione peroxidise and coenzyme Q10. These pass their electron burden down the line to second-line antioxidants, such as vitamins A and E and eventually to vitamin C.

Vitamin B12 in high doses helps to quench this pro-inflammatory fire and I suspect that this explains why high-dose injections are so helpful in so many disease processes. The benefits of B12 are not predicted by blood tests – since B12 has no toxicity the decision to use is a clinical one based on clinical need.

TESTS FOR INFLAMMATION

Tests which indicate inflammation in the body include:
- C-reactive protein
- Plasma viscosity and erythrocyte sedimentation rate (ESR)

However, these are not very sensitive and do not, for example, flag up the low-grade inflammation in arteries which results in arteriosclerosis.

Inflammation for healing and repair

Inflammation is necessary to heal and repair tissue damage. In the short term, we see all the classical symptoms of inflammation – pain, heat, swelling, redness and loss of function. We see this in patients who have undergone surgery – the wound-site is initially inflamed, then the immune system lays down fibrous tissue, initially in a rather disorganised way, as a sticking plaster which leaves a thickened line along the site of the cut; this then toughens up over the course of some days, but in the longer term re-models to leave a patch that is almost as good as new, but often a small scar remains.

Inflammation occurs in all tissues, such as:

- **Arteries** – Due to damage from turbulent blood flow, high blood sugar and toxic stress from noxious gases or toxic metals. It results in atherosclerotic plaques, which of course cause problems in their own right because they further narrow the blood vessel.
- **Joints** – This can result in excessive growth of bone or connective material, which may pinch nerves and cause other such mechanical problems. We call these 'osteophytes'.
- **The gut** – Inflammation in the gut may result in adhesions forming between loops of the intestines, which may cause obstruction subsequently.
- **The lining of the womb** in response to infection – This can narrow the fallopian tubes and result in infertility.
- **The lungs** as a result of irritation from, say, cigarette smoking or industrial pollution – This means that the lungs become stiff and thickened and lose their elasticity and their ability to exchange respiratory gases. Sufferers develop emphysema and are called 'pink puffers'.
- **The liver** – Resulting in fatty liver disease and cirrhosis. Indeed, we are seeing an epidemic of non-alcoholic fatty liver disease due to Western diets high in sugar and refined carbohydrates.
- **The pancreas** – We know many cases of pancreatitis are due to poor antioxidant status.

So inflammation as a tool of healing and repair is a vital sticking plaster in the short term but carries potential dangers in the long term. It is the old story – prevention is better than cure. If one can identify and avoid causes of damage, whether that be mechanical or inflammatory (infection, allergy or autoimmunity), and therefore the further inflammation that follows, our bodies are going to last very much longer.

TESTS OF CELL DAMAGE

Cell-free DNA – DNA should be found only within the nucleus of each cell. In measuring DNA which is not packaged up within a cell, this test therefore shows the level of cell damage – any DNA lying outside must derive from a severely damaged cell.

TESTS FOR INFLAMMATION

Body temperature – Running a fever is symptomatic of generalised inflammation. However, with age one's ability to do such declines as energy delivery mechanisms decline.

Erythrocyte sedimentation rate (ESR)

Plasma viscosity

C-reactive protein

Gut inflammation (faecal calprotectin) – This is typically raised in inflammatory bowel disease. It may also turn out to be a better screening test for bowel cancers than looking for blood in the stool.

However, with mild inflammation all the above tests may be normal. Indeed, inflammation is so much a part of Western diets and lifestyles that the normal ranges for all the above have been cranked upwards. The normal range for ESR used to be up to 10 mm/hour; now it is 20 mm/hour, increasing with age.

Inflammation to fight infection

The microbe (germ) is nothing. The terrain (milieu) is everything.

LOUIS PASTEUR (1822–1896)

The human body is a potential free lunch for microbes. Microbes are survivors – we can never eliminate them. Humans must live in equilibrium with them. They coat all surfaces, from skin and gut to vagina and ears. Indeed, we all have our own personal, unique spectrum of microbes, which can be used, like DNA fingerprinting, to identify individuals. It is hard work for microbes to scrape a living on surfaces – they are always trying for the richer meal contained below. If they succeed we become infected, quickly develop septicaemia and succumb.

Think of infection as the arms race.

The first line of defence against infection is avoidance. This starts with good Public Health measures. Throughout history, cholera has killed more people than any other disease. The rate of infectious disease fell rapidly in Britain when the Victorians developed a system of pressurised water supply that ran above the sewers. This fall long preceded vaccination. Good housing and clean foods are equally important. The point here is that if any person gets a sufficient dose of a sufficiently aggressive pathogen, then they will succumb.

It has become an accepted part of growing up that we should travel and enjoy multiple sexual partners, but this carries great risk of infection. Any healthy person can pick up HIV, hepatitis, chlamydia, herpes, tetanus, malaria and so on. I advise my CFS patients not to travel to exotic locations and be wary of vaccination because it often makes them ill.

A further line of defence is taste and smell, and learning through experience and intuition. This is important not just for the obvious infection and poisons, but also allergy.

SKIN – AN ESSENTIAL BARRIER

Skin provides a physical barrier. It therefore needs to be intact – cuts and breakages need to be kept clean. All surfaces and defences (skin, ears, tears, saliva, urine) are slightly acidic and microbes are acid sensitive. I do not advocate disinfectants and antiseptic soaps – we have colonies of friendly bacteria on the skin that live in a happy symbiosis with us and physically displace the pathogens. Indeed, everyday exposures to dirt are helpful to keep the immune system on its toes.

STOMACH ACID

The stomach provides an acid defence. Day-to-day microbial attack comes either from foods eaten or microbes inhaled. Those inhaled microbes become stuck onto the sticky mucus lining the nose and lungs where cilia sweep them up to the throat for swallowing. They should descend into a bath of stomach acid, where they are destroyed. An acid stomach is a vital defence. Any amount of acid is helpful. The initial viral or bacterial load determines the severity of an infection because there is certain inertia in the immune system – it takes time to ramp up its defences and during this time microbial numbers can build up quickly. Given the right substrate, bacteria can double their numbers every 20 minutes. So a small 'loading dose' of microbes gives more time for the immune system to swing into action.

Hypochlorrhydria (low stomach acid) is common in my CFS patients and, I suspect, a major risk factor for the condition. These patients often have a history of tendency to food poisoning and gut viruses (like Epstein Barr, coxsackie B, cytomegalovirus) as well as upper fermenting gut with other microbes. Pancreatic enzymes and bile salts are also toxic to microbes. Quick digestion and absorption of food reduces upper gut fermentation and infection.

ANTI-MICROBIAL DIET

Diet is critical. Fat is Nature's way of tucking fuel out of the way of microbes. Microbes cannot ferment fat. How do I know this? Because I can leave a lump of lard in my fridge for weeks and it does not go off – ditto a bottle of olive oil in my pantry. Western diets are high in sugar and carbohydrates that are readily fermented by microbes, so microbe numbers may be high in the upper gut.

Vegetables are rich in fibre, or 'prebiotics', which feed the friendly bacteria, but it's not quite as easy as you think – so-called 'friendly' microbes are perfectly capable of invading the body and causing peritonitis and septicaemia. However, since microbes are unavoidable (and some are helpful), antibiotics are not the answer as we would then kill the helpful bacteria as well. One policy of the arms race is to tackle this by competing for space and substrate by eating high-dose probiotics. By increasing the numbers of good bacteria this crowds out the unwanted microbes. We can easily grow these in our kitchens by making yoghurts and sauerkrauts. Kefir, for example, contains a combination of bacteria that kill yeast.

If you look at life from the point of view of a plant, it too does not want to be eaten by microbes. Fresh plant material is rich in natural anti-microbials, all of which help to reduce microbial numbers. Deep-rooting perennial plants are likely to be richer in such – we should become good cooks and take advantage of herbs, spices, nuts and seeds, all of which are difficult to ferment and contain natural anti-microbials and antioxidants.

GUT WALL PROTECTION

The gut wall itself is protected by various molecules that make microbes less sticky – so they cannot get a foothold and are washed out. These include:

- **Mucous** – As Dr David Freed, consultant immunologist, used to enjoy saying, 'It may be snot to you, but it's my bread and butter!'
- **Secretory IgA** – Large amounts are poured onto all surfaces (gut, skin, tears, saliva) to kill microbes.
- **Defensins** – These are sulphur-containing proteins which kill microbes directly. Interestingly they also form a cobweb-like matrix which lines the gut and prevents microbes getting too close to the absorptive surface. I do not know how to boost defensin production – yet!
- **Lactoferrin** – Microbes are greedy for micronutrients, especially iron. Binding up iron to get it out of the metabolic way is an essential defence. Breast milk is high in lactoferrin and helps to protect the immature gut of the newborn baby from infection.

The overwhelming majority of microbes are dealt with by the above defence mechanisms. The vital feature of these innate defences is that they do not involve inflammation. The immune system is the last resort. This is because once the immune system has been activated, we risk the problem of friendly fire. Many, if not most, disease processes, from cancer and auto-immunity to arthritis and irritable bowel, are infection driven – either directly or indirectly, through an inappropriate switching on of inflammation. Avoiding infection by interventions to support our innate defences is a vital part of long-term good health.

Allergy and autoimmunity – useless inflammation

Evolution intended for us to be bred, born and brought up in the same place, inheriting our mother's gut flora, eating locally grown food and sniffing local plants and animals, in a chemically clean environment. Soon after birth and weaning we would have been exposed to very few, if any, 'new' antigens. The occasional traveller might bring a new virus, but the immune system would have been exposed daily to familiarity, learned the status quo and behaved appropriately.

Problems arise when the immune system gets its wires crossed. This is a forgivable offence – it has a very difficult job to do. It has to distinguish potential goodies from potential baddies. At the molecular level they all look pretty similar – lumps of DNA, membranes, proteins, and other cellular material. Indeed, some authorities believe that nearly 50 per cent of so-called human DNA is in fact viral DNA. Furthermore, where there is tissue damage the immune system is responsible for clearing things up.

The problem with Western lifestyles is that the immune system faces massive new challenges. We eat a wider range of foods than ever before, and are exposed to many new microbes and to many different and novel plant antigens.

A major problem comes from chemicals. Chemicals twist familiar antigens in unrecognisable ways so the immune system 'smells' them differently. Some chemicals have the potential to switch on the immune system; we call these adjuvants. In order of importance, I suspect (based on research and clinical experience) these adjuvants are:

Infection – Viruses, bacteria and yeasts. Many of my CFS patients are post-infectious. Increasing sexual promiscuity, the world population rise and travel are all problems.

Vaccinations – These are designed to switch the immune system on through using chemical adjuvants. Dead or attenuated microbes injected into the body are recognised as such by the immune system – non-threatening. For vaccinations to be effective they need an immune system wake-up call – usually a heavy metal, such as mercury or aluminium. In the past silicones were used. More recently a toxic fat squalene has been employed. When that switching on of the immune system is desirable we call it immunity. It can be very helpful. However, I have seen many autistic children whose disease followed vaccination, ditto CFS, auto-immunity and dementia.

Chemical pollution of the environment – A study in Japan showed that hay fever was more common in the city that the countryside despite pollen counts being lower in the city. The answer for this apparent anomaly was diesel particulates from vehicle exhausts. Chemicals stick to antigens and change their shape so they become more foreign and unrecognisable by the immune system. Our immune systems are racist! The presence of foreign materials, be these chemicals, microbes or tissue transplants, means they must launch an attack.

The Pill and HRT – These increase the risk of autoimmunity. I suspect this explains why autoimmunity is much more common in women than men currently. This may be because of its immunosuppressive effects which allow infections to flourish.

Molecular mimicry – This is one mechanism by which autoimmunity may be switched on. The idea here is that the body makes antibodies against foods or microbes which then, through sheer chance, cross-react with the body's own molecules. So, for example, ankylosing spondylitis is thought to be caused by molecular mimicry. Antibodies are made against *Klebsiella* bacteria in the gut which then cross-react with spinal ligaments. (One has to be a particular tissue type for this to happen – namely, HLA B27 positive). There is some evidence to suggest that rheumatoid arthritis may be partly due to molecular mimicry between the gut bacterium *Proteus mirabilis* and tissue types HLA DR1 and 4. Clinically one sometimes sees arthritis following viral infections (palindromic rheumatism) and this too may be molecular mimicry.

Allergy such as gluten sensitivity may result in autoimmune thyroid disease.

AUTOIMMUNE ASSOCIATIONS HAVE BEEN SHOWN BETWEEN:

- Epstein-Barr virus (EBV) and genotype HLA DR-15 (puts one at risk of multiple sclerosis)
- EBV and HLA DR3 (puts one at risk of autoimmune thyroiditis)
- EBV and HLA DR4 (puts one at risk of autoimmune cardiomyopathy)
- EBV and HLA DR7 (puts one at risk of primary biliary cirrhosis)
- EBV and HLA DR7 plus smoking (puts one at risk of rheumatoid arthritis and multiple sclerosis)

In addition:

- EBV has been associated with 33 autoimmune diseases, including systemic lupus erythematosis and Sjogren's syndrome.
- CMV (cytomegalovirus) has also been associated with autoimmune reactions.
- Streptococcal throat infections used to result in rheumatic fever – oddly less so nowadays.
- Guttate psoriasis may be switched on by a streptococcal sore throat.
- *Helicobacter pylori* infection is associated with idiopathic thrombocytopenic purpura (ITP), systemic sclerosis, Crohn's disease, Guillain-Barre syndrome and other vasculitic conditions. Eradication of *H. pylori* has resulted in resolution of ITP and also anti-phospholipid syndrome, BUT *H. pylori* infection is protective for childhood asthma.
- Wegener's granulomatosis may be switched on by *Staphlococci* in the nose.
- Antibodies against yeast – namely, ASCA (anti-saccharomyces cerevisiae antibody) – are predictive of developing Crohn's disease.
- ASCA (antibody against yeast) is associated with arteriosclerosis – this too may be an autoimmune disease.
- Vaccinations increase the risk of autoimmunity – for example, swine 'flu vaccination has been followed by epidemics of Guillain-Barre syndrome and narcolepsy.
- Parasitic worms are protective against many forms of autoimmunity. They have a proven track record in protecting against inflammatory bowel disease.

Autoimmunity now affects 1 in 20 Westerners. We should be taking active steps to avoid it because it is much more difficult to switch off than on.

2. The emotional hole in the energy pot

The brain weighs 2 per cent of body weight but at rest consumes 20 per cent of all energy produced. In other words, it is enormously demanding of energy. Some people have a constitutionally high level of anxiety and this punches an emotional hole in their energy bucket. Being anxious is exhausting. Had such highly strung characters lived 10,000 years ago they would have been the sentries at the opening to the tribe's cave. They would have heard a sabre-toothed tiger fart a mile away. By contrast I would have been snoring my way through the night. By day the sentries would have been exhausted, but no matter – the good sleepers would have gone hunting to feed the tribe.

Hypervigilance

Hyper-vigilance is a great drainer of energy. Sometimes people are born hyper-vigilant; sometimes it is acquired. Childhood abuse is a major risk factor for CFS.

Hyper-vigilance and anxiety disturb sleep, so there is less time for healing and repair to take place.

There are a great many psychological techniques that are extremely helpful in treating, or coping with, the psychological causes of hyper-vigilance. However, whatever those techniques are, they require energy for two reasons. Firstly, one needs energy to drive the mental processes to make the necessary psychological changes. Secondly, ATP is not just the energy molecule; it is essential for other neurotransmitters to be effective. It is a necessary co-transmitter for many neuro-transmitters. Tackling all the energy delivery issues has profoundly positive effects on mood and psychological health and greatly enhances the benefit of psychotherapy.

The fermenting brain

A further mechanism by which neurotransmitters may be wasted has to do with the fermenting gut. Professor Nishihara has demonstrated that fermenting microbes in the gut may also be present in the brain, with the potential to ferment neurotransmitters to LSD and amphetamine-like substances, and who knows what else? These microbes may additionally interfere with energy delivery mechanisms in the brain. Regardless of the mechanism, this makes sense of the long-recognised clinical link between gut and brain disorders. Correcting gut function may help plug the emotional hole in the brain energy pot.

C. Mechanical problems: structure, friction and wear and tear – allergic joints, connective tissue and muscles

Structure

Humans are probably at greater risk of mechanical damage than any other mammal because relatively recently in evolution we chose to walk around on two legs. This brought evolutionary advantages – humans are not the fastest predator, but they can run great distances without fatigue and wear down their prey. Their arms and shoulders were freed up so they could throw spears and rocks. This made them excellent hunters. In a mammal Olympics, humans would win the marathon and the javelin competitions. Cheetahs would win the 100-metres sprint.

However, a vertebral column that evolved to work from the horizontal now has to function in the vertical position. This it achieves marvellously so long as all else is well. The vertebral column is inherently unstable and what keeps it functioning well and pain free is a powerful system of muscles and connective tissue which holds it in place. There are many wonderful mechanical interventions to help us achieve this most efficiently, but discussion of these is outside the scope of this book. As a clinical doctor, I tend to look at the body from the point of view of essential organs like the brain, gut and heart, but osteopaths take the opposite view – the body is a physical machine with brain, gut and heart merely the supporting staff. Get the structural aspects right and everything else falls into line. A great deal of athletic training has to do with correct posture and there are very few people who would not benefit from such training.

Most people stand incorrectly. Furthermore, if we injure ourselves enough to cause pain we will adjust our posture to deal with that in the short term. This may well leave us with even worse posture. Within the brain we have a three-dimensional map of how the body should be and this is maintained by the fabulous cerebellum, which is responsible for balance and posture. Each muscle has to be set at just the right degree of tension to hold us in place. I suspect that many of the subtle manipulative techniques, such as Bowen therapy, or Reiki healing, which cannot be explained by simple mechanical means, could be explained by a re-mapping of the brain. It may be that there are learned muscle spasms that may in the short term be in response to pain, but in the long term cause pain in their own right, which could be re-mapped by appropriate techniques to afford relief. Whatever the explanation, there has to be one, because I see so many people benefit from these techniques for which modern medicine appears to have no good explanation. It may be hard work but remember Ovid: 'exitus acta probat' (the end justifies the deed). I often see people whose health has been restored simply through attention to posture and exercise.

Friction, and wear and tear

Friction is damaging. It results in wear and tear, and is energy sapping. All moving machines use tricks to minimise friction, such as finely engineered weight-bearing surfaces, ball bearings and lubricating oils. The body is no different and employs similar techniques. These include the ultra-smooth surfaces of joints, synovial lubricating fluid within joints, special pockets of such fluid to minimise the friction of moving tendons (bursae) and a softer matrix of fibrous/elastic material we call collagen. This is further steeped in a semi-solid colloidal, mucous matrix. Collectively we call this the connective tissue – a terribly boring name for a divine conglomeration that allows our soft tissues to look gorgeous and function beautifully despite being suspended from an unforgiving skeleton. Indeed, there is a seamless transition from rock-hard bone into soft pliable muscles and internal organs via these tough tendons and elastic tissue. Furthermore, this is a mass of electrical charges which give just the right degree of stickiness – not so much that skin hangs down, but sufficient to allow tissues to glide smoothly over each other and not so much that a limb seizes solid. In addition, this stickiness must be absolutely uniform through the tissues, otherwise areas of relative stiffness would concentrate the lines of force, and concentrations of such are painful. We call these by many names, including fibrositis, rheumatics, spondylitis, lumbago, screws, rheumatics, bursitis, tendonitis, fasciitis, repetitive strain injury, stiff neck and others.

An understanding of the magnificent properties of connective tissue explains why so many different therapies are effective. This includes TENS, acupuncture, massage therapy, magnets and manipulative treatments such as osteopathy, shiatsu, McTimoney chiropractic and many others. We know these treatments are effective because they are so widely used by patients who get relief. Again remember Ovid!

Raw materials to heal and repair

Where wear and tear has taken place we need raw materials and energy to repair. This is dependent on good diet and gut function, good energy delivery for the repair to take place and good sleep to allow time for repair to be effected. We get less good at all these things this as we age. As it's said, old age does not come alone – but it does not have to!

Increasing friction causes the symptom of stiffness

If the rate of wear and tear exceeds the rate of healing and repair then there will be progressive damage. Friction builds up initially, resulting in a sensation of stiffness as the body tries to protect itself from itself. Sometimes one can feel a grating/fine vibration, or even hear the friction, a creaking noise, where there is a bursitis or tendonitis. If friction is ignored, further damage will result in inflammation and all the problems that accompany such. Indeed, inflammation will further complicate the clinical picture and allergy and auto-immunity come into play – lots of potential for vicious cycles here.

Allergic joints, muscles and connective tissue

Allergy never ceases to surprise and amaze me for the multiplicity of symptoms that it can cause. It is clear to me that any part of the body can react with allergy. Indeed, one of my mentors, Dr Honor Anthony, used to say that most arthritis was allergy. During the 1980s I was not sure. Now I know – allergy is a big player. Sometimes one is lucky and the answer is a simple food allergy. However, increasingly I am seeing that allergy to gut microbes is a major factor. The best example of this is ankylosing spondilitis. This was worked out by Dr Alan Ebringer[7] of the Middlesex Hospital as a case of molecular mimicry, whereby the immune system gets its wires crossed. The idea here is that the gut contains bacteria, *Klebsiella*, which the immune system may make antibodies to. If it just so happens that you have a particular tissue type (HLA B27), then the microscopic shape of the spinal ligaments is sufficiently similar to *Klebsiella* to allow cross-reaction. Antibodies meant for *Klebsiella* start to stick to spinal ligaments and switch on inflammation. Inflammation of the ligaments of the spine causes the symptoms of ankylosing spondylitis (AS). Ebringer did further work suggesting that rheumatoid arthritis was allergy to *Proteus mirabilis* bacteria. Psoriatic arthritis may be allergy to yeast because so many sufferers respond well to anti-yeast regimes.

The mechanism by which allergy is switched on

What I suspect happens is that joints, connective tissue and muscle becomes sensitised as a result of mechanical damage. Tearing or bruising means that these connective tissues come in direct contact with blood, which may be carrying food antigens or antigens of fermenting microbes. I suspect the allergy is switched on at that time and the pain which follows the muscle damage and which persists long term is mis-attributed to damage, when actually it is allergy. So a torn muscle in the back from, say, lifting a heavy load could sensitise to, say, dairy products and it is the consumption of dairy subsequently which keeps the problem on the boil. I have three patients whose allergic toe (bunion) settled down through avoiding dairy products.

The clinical picture of joint pain or connective tissue pain is usually obvious. However, I increasingly see the allergic muscle which produces a severe cramp-like pain.

D. Growth promotion

Benign and malignant growths (cancer)

Growths of some sort are an inevitable result of modern Western diets and lifestyles. We are seeing epidemics of benign breast lumps, polycystic ovarian disease, skin lumps and nodules, neuromas, fibromas, thyroid lumps, prostate hypertrophy and so on. Benign lumps appear to increase the risk of malignant lumps so any such should be seen as an early warning symptom. Benign lumps arise because of growth-promoting factors in modern Western diets and lifestyles. The main growth promoters are:

- Sugar (and refined carbohydrates)
- Insulin
- Oestrogen and progesterone (the Pill and HRT)
- Dairy products (These also make people tall and fat and these too are risk factors.)
- Growth hormone mimics – organochlorine pesticides (very persistent in fat)

A cancer may result when there is growth promotion on top of genetic damage. For a cancer to develop, there are two clear and separate steps – firstly DNA has to be damaged faster than it can be repaired. DNA is constantly being damaged by, for example, background radiation. Happily we have enzymes, such as DNA repair and DNA ligase, which spend their lives trotting up and down DNA, cutting out the damaged sections and repairing them. But if the rate of damage exceeds the rate of repair, then DNA will be permanently damaged, with the potential to block genes or activate them. If a gene involved with cell replication is affected then uncontrolled cell division may occur – that is, an early cancer. The second step is that these uncontrolled cells have to grow and this will be enhanced by growth promoters, as listed above. Even tall people have a greater risk of cancer because cancer is a result of processes having to do with growth. This means that cancer is multi-factorial and several causal threads are involved. These include:

- Damage to DNA by toxic stress, such as POPs (persistent organic pollutants)
- Damage to DNA by free radicals from inflammation
- Micronutrient deficiencies resulting in poor ability to heal and repair DNA

- Micronutrient deficiencies resulting in poor antioxidant function
- Poor energy delivery systems resulting in a switch to anaerobic metabolism which creates an environment favourable to cancer cells

Followed by:
- Growth promoters (as listed above)
- Growth hormone mimics

Once a diagnosis of cancer has been given, this means that there will be trillions of cancer cells already established. For a tumour to be visible on a scan, there must be between a thousand million and a million million cells present. Anything that can be done to reduce this total load is going to be helpful. Standard conventional approaches to cancer – that is, surgery, radiotherapy and chemotherapy – all have their place. The problem is targeting treatment so that as much of the tumour is killed as possible with normal cells spared. In practice this is a very difficult balancing act.

However, there are other things that can be done over and above the conventional approaches which not only make these treatments more effective, but greatly reduce side effects. In my experience and evidence from a large body of medical literature, these interventions improve the chances of survival.

The fundamental principles behind these extra therapies are as follows:

- Starve the growth of its food supply – that is, sugar and refined carbohydrates.
- Get rid of growth promoters – female sex hormones, dairy, insulin (through diet).
- Ensure excellent nutritional status with vitamins and minerals (to allow healing and repair).
- Consume vitamin C to bowel tolerance.
- Improve antioxidant status (to mop up free radicals created by the cancer treatments and limit side effects).
- Sleep well (as that is when healing and repair take place).
- Do a good detox regime (to get rid of exogenous tumour initiators and growth promoters).
- Exercise.
- Reduce inflammation.
- Address energy delivery mechanisms.
- Use natural anti-cancer substances.
- Monitor the effects of treatment.

Prion disorders

Alzheimer's disease, Parkinson's disease and CJD are all prion disorders. Motor neurone disease may or may not be one also.

Cancers, of course, are immortal cells which replicate themselves and build up to cause problems. Viruses are strips of DNA which replicate themselves and build up in the body to cause problems. I think of prion disorders as **protein cancers**. Prions are proteins which are normally present in the body and perform essential functions. However, if they come into contact with a particular toxin or heavy metal, or another twisted prion (rotten apple effect), then they too twist and distort. They twist in such a way that they cannot be broken down by the body's enzyme systems and effectively become immortal. Difficulties arise because they obstruct normal biochemistry so cells malfunction. Pathologically this is known as **amyloid**.

Although amyloid can occur anywhere in the body, the biggest problem is in the brain. This is perhaps partly because the brain is a closed box and therefore there is no room for all this excess protein to be dumped, and partly because each part of the brain is vital and any loss of function is quickly noticed.

These protein cancers cause problems which may take many years to become apparent and so far there are no known methods of slowing down this process.

From work done with BSE ('mad cow disease', which is also a protein cancer like CJD), there appear to be two phases. After the build-up of prions, there then appears to be an autoimmune phase, where the body suddenly recognises this protein as being foreign. This causes inflammation against the prion material in an attempt to get rid of it, but the inflammation does far more damage than the prion and the disease process is suddenly accelerated. In BSE this is often triggered by a stressful event, such as a calving or very cold weather.

Huntington's disease fits many of the criteria for a prion disorder so the approach to treatment would be similar to any other.

What creates prions?

Just as cancers have triggers and causes, we now recognise some of the triggers for prion disorders. The best documented are heavy metals, pesticides and natural toxins, but there may well be others. For example:

- **Alzheimer's disease** has been linked to aluminium toxicity (as, for example, in dialysis dementia) and also mercury toxicity. The Mad Hatter in *Alice in Wonderland* was mercury poisoned – mercury was used in the hat-making process at that time. Mercury may be coming from dental amalgam fillings. Both mercury and aluminium have been, or continue to be, used in vaccinations. The prion protein is **amyloid beta protein**.

- **Parkinson's disease** is associated with manganese toxicity and organophosphate pesticides. The prion protein involved is **alpha synuclein**.
- **CJD:** Studies of BSE show clear association with exposure to organophosphate pesticides and also to manganese (in the absence of copper). Human cases of CJD are more likely to be related either to pesticide poisoning or direct infection through vaccination, blood transfusion or surgery. I think it highly unlikely that CJD may be acquired by eating beef. The prion protein involved is **PrPSc**.
- **Motor neurone disease** is also associated with manganese poisoning and cycad (a natural toxin from beans).

Energy delivery is involved in prion disorders (problems with mitochondria, thyroid and adrenal function) and, indeed, correction of such may be a vital part of treatment. (Mitochondria are the power stations in each cell; glucose is converted into energy within them, in the presence of oxygen.)

E. Genetics

Genetics have been blamed for a great many ills. However, the World Health Organisation tells us that the majority of problems arise from gene-environment interactions – that is to say, if the environment can be put right, then the gene problem can be overcome. So, for example, I see many patients with CFS and a central player here is poor mitochondrial function. Mitochondria have their own genes, which are different from the cell's own genomic DNA. However, if that gene defect happens to be related to a problem with endogenous production of coenzyme Q10, then that can be fixed simply by administering coenzyme Q10. Indeed, I am coming to the view that as we age we all become less good at producing coenzyme Q10 and maybe we should all be taking a supplement of 100–300 mg daily in order to protect our mitochondria and slow the ageing process.

Just because a patient has a genetic lesion does not mean nothing can be done for them. Dr Henry Turkel specialised in treating Down's syndrome. Many of his patients were hypothyroid (they were not producing enough thyroxin for their metabolisms to work at the right pace). Correction of this together with diets and other standard techniques of nutritional medicine resulted in patients functioning at a higher physical and intellectual level.[8]

TEST: SNPS

Single nucleotide polymorphisms, or SNPs (pronounced 'snips'), can be tested for. These are the most common type of genetic variation among people. Identifying SNPs may indicate susceptibility to certain diseases. However, I never do this test – it is rather expensive and rarely has implications for management.

Acquired genetic lesions

I am extremely fortunate to be able to work very closely with Dr John McLaren-Howard of Acumen Laboratories, who is the most brilliant biochemist. His brilliance arises because he applies cutting-edge technology to clinical problems. A most useful test that he makes available is **DNA adducts**. This is a measure of what is stuck onto DNA. Of course, DNA should be pristine – it is the genetic blueprint. Having something stuck on to it (such as a toxic metal, pesticide or volatile organic compound) is bad news for obvious reasons – the genetic code cannot be accurately read. Furthermore, Acumen can identify which gene the adduct is stuck on to; this may block this gene or activate it – both are undesirable because normal gene expression is upset.

Acumen goes on to do further analysis using a technique called **microarray**. This allows a more detailed view of DNA and how it is expressed. This brings us on to epigenetics – the DNA may be intact but one cannot get at it, perhaps because of poor methylation (the biochemical tool we need to start and finish reading DNA – page 200). We need this biochemical tool to start and to finish reading DNA.

Summary

Modern Western lifestyles are very damaging to DNA because of the pernicious combination of toxic stress, micronutrient deficiencies and inflammation. With Acumen Laboratories' tests we can prove this is so. Using sustainable, ecological medicine we can prevent and treat.

CHAPTER 3

The tools of the trade to correct and treat mechanisms of disease

Life is really simple, but we insist on making it complicated.

CONFUCIUS (c. 551–479 BC)

Introduction

The tools of the trade divide quite neatly into two sections: first, those we should all be doing all the time, in order to reduce the possibility of ill health arising in the first place, and then, second, the 'bolt-on' extras which should be employed where a specific condition has been identified. What follows below is a checklist for each of these two sections and thereafter the reader will find more detail on each in the two sub-sections.

1. The Basic Package –
what we should all be doing all the time

To keep healthy we should:
- A. Eat a **Paleo-ketogenic** diet (staple foods: meat, fish, eggs, vegetables, nuts, seeds, salad, berries; occasional treats: dairy, grains, fruit).
- B. Take **supplementary multivitamins**, minerals and essential fatty acids.
- C. Get the correct amount of **sleep**.
- D. **Exercise**.
- E. Get plenty of **sunshine** and **daylight**.
- F. Reduce the **chemical burden**.
- G. Have sufficient physical and mental **security** to satisfy our universal need to love and care, and be loved and cared for.
- H. **Avoid infections** and treat any that arise aggressively.

2. The bolt-on extras – the therapeutic tools of the trade

We do not have all the tools to treat all the problems, but the body is fabulous at healing itself. We only have to get the package 51 per cent right and the body will do the rest. Only 49 per cent right and one is on the slippery downhill slope. Many tools multi-task. For example, ATP is the energy molecule and a neurotransmitter. Also, high-dose vitamin B12 may be used to improve mitochondrial function, for detoxing via the methylation cycle, as an antioxidant and for its anti-inflammatory properties by damping down the pro-inflammatory fire of the NO/ON/OO cycle (see page 220). In summary, these tools are:

I. Tools to treat acute infections (page 89)
II. Tools to treat poor energy delivery:
   a. Mitochondrial function – the engines that make energy (see page 90)
   b. Thyroid function – the accelerator pedal (see page 93)
   c. Adrenal function – the gear box
   d. Circadian rhythms – timing is vital
III. Tools to treat inflammatory conditions:
   a. Tools to help to damp down the pro-inflammatory biochemical fire of the NO/ON/OO cycle:
      i. Allergen avoidance
      ii. Correct antioxidant status
      iii. Vitamin D
      iv. Vitamin B12
      v. Alkalinisation – magnesium carbonate
      vi. Low-dose naltrexone
      vii. Exercise, music, singing, love and laughter
   b. De-sensitising techniques to turn off allergies:
      i. Enzyme-potentiated desensitisation and neutralisation
      ii. Oral immunotherapy – switching off food allergy with low-dose foods
      iii. Homeopathy
IV. Tools to improve gut function:
   a. Reduce numbers of bacteria and yeast in the mouth
   b. Low/zero carbohydrate ketogenic diets
   c. Improve digestion: acid supplements, digestive enzymes, bile salts
   d. Probiotics
   e. Transdermal supplements
   f. Vitamin C

1. The Basic Package

A. Paleo-ketogenic diet

> *The Cure is in the Kitchen.*
>
> DR SHERRY ROGERS, environmental physician

I spend more time talking about diet than all other subjects put together. Changing one's diet is the most difficult but perhaps the most important thing one needs to do for good health. Anyone eating a modern Western diet high in sugar and refined carbohydrates can expect to become fat, feel fatigued and die prematurely from heart disease, cancer or dementia.

People initially complain that the Paleo-ketogenic diet is boring. Actually, it is far more varied in composition, texture and flavour than any contemporary Western diet as these actually rely on remarkably few foods – and a lot of artificial flavouring. What gets in the way is addiction – people subconsciously recognise the addictive hit they get from high carbohydrate diets and mistake the absence of this for boredom. The convenience of modern Western diets is also a major factor.

There is no one-size-fits-all Paleo-ketogenic diet, but general principles that need to be honed to individual needs. The basic diet is as below, but changes may need to be made if there are allergies to foods or problems with the fermenting gut.

Allowed foods

- **Meat:** Choose from chicken, beef, lamb, pork, turkey, duck and 'game' meats, such as venison, pheasant, rabbit and so on. Liver, kidney and offal generally are excellent foods. Fatty meat is ideal and tastes wonderful! Use preserved meats such as bacon, ham and salami in moderation and try to avoid nitrates and nitrites – they do not all contain these.
- **Eggs:** These are an excellent source of lecithin (eat soft yolks).
- **Fish:** Choose especially from salmon, mackerel, cod, haddock. (Take care with smoked fish which often contains dyes). Tinned fish in brine or olive oil is fine.
- **Shellfish,** including tinned shrimps, prawns, mussels, cockles, etc.
- **Green vegetables**.
- **Salad vegetables,** including avocado, lettuce, tomato, cucumber, celery, peppers, onion, cress, bamboo shoots, mushrooms.
- **Olive, nut and seed oils,** such as sunflower, olive, sesame, grapeseed, hemp, linseed, rape.
- **Spices and herbs,** including chilli, cumin, ginger, coriander, pepper, cloves.
- **Fermented foods** are ideal – for example, kefir fermented on soya, coconut, almond or rice milk.
- **French dressing** – make your own from olive oil, lemon juice, garlic, mustard.
- **Salt** – this needs to be added to a true Paleo-ketogenic diet; suggest sea salt 4 grams (a teaspoon is about 5 grams) daily.

It is vital to recognise that we need to power our bodies with fat – firstly, medium-chain fats – that is, animal fat (lard), coconut oil, cocoa butter fat. Butter is an excellent fat so long as there is no dairy allergy. Eat these medium-chain fats in abundance to fuel your body and brain – in particular, the brain is in need of these. Secondly, we need short-chain fatty acids from the fermentation of vegetable fibre. Vegetable fibre and prebiotics are fermented by friendly bacteroides in the lower gut to short-chain fatty acids. Indeed, these ferment to produce n-butyrate to fuel the lining of the large bowel directly. Absence of bacteroides results in major gut pathology.

We also need fats as building materials for cell membranes. These are the long-chain fatty acids (vegetable, nut, seed and fish oils). The ideal proportion of omega-6 to omega-3 fats is four to one. Hemp oil is very close to this.

Fermented foods are excellent because the carbohydrate content has been fermented out and gut friendly microbes grow. Sauerkraut is an example of a fermented vegetable. Kefir can be used to ferment nut or bean milks and is very easy to work with – one starter lasts a lifetime since new cultures can be grown from previous ones.

The following foods are low in carbohydrates. With a serious ferment-ing gut even they may need to be avoided but most people can eat them without problems:

- **Dark chocolate:** at least 70 per cent cocoa solids
- **Berries:** avoid high-sugar fruits and fruit juices which are as dangerous, arguably more so, than table sugar
- **Seeds:** sunflower, poppy, sesame
- **Nuts:** peanut, Brazil, hazel, cashew, pistachio, walnut, etc; nut butter spreads, tahini (sesame seed spread)
- **Pulses:** when cooked, these are rich in starches and vegetable fibre; the latter is excellent, but some people will ferment the starch in pulses and suffer bloating; this is a good indication to address the fermenting gut (page 201)
- Some young people with excellent gut function, no allergies and no fermenting gut may be able to tolerate modest amounts of whole grains.

Remember 'fats good, carbs bad' as the source of energy.

Allowed drinks

- **Bottled water** (ideal) or filtered water (second best). When water is lost during hot weather or athletic performance, or gastroenteritis, additional minerals should be taken. My standard recipe is 1 gram of my multi-mineral mix (see below) with 2 grams of salt in 1 litre of water taken ad lib.
- **Herbal teas:** redbush, rosehip tea, peppermint, etc.
- **Tea and coffee** in moderation are fine so long as caffeine is tolerated.

Principles of a healthy diet

In order of importance, the aspects of modern Western diet and gut function which commonly cause symptoms – from irritable bowel syndrome to fatigue – and disease – from metabolic syndrome to cancer and dementia – are:

- Sugar, refined carbohydrate, fruit and fruit sugar – which are addictive, convenient and cheap.
- Fermentation of these carbohydrates in the upper gut by unfriendly microbes – very common in modern Westerners. Live, actively fermenting probiotics, such as kefir, help to protect against this problem.
- Insufficient fat – we have been brainwashed into believing fat is bad. Meat fat is the perfect fuel for our tiny guts.
- Lack of micronutrients in food because of modern agricultural techniques.
- Allergy to foods – most commonly to grains and dairy products.
- Toxins in the diet – such as colourings, flavourings, artificial sweeteners, pesticide residues, plasticiser residues.
- Burnt fats – friendly oils and fats can be twisted into unfriendly trans-fats by heat and hydrogenation. (The latter is the technique for making margarine.)
- Socially acceptable addictions in excess (alcohol, caffeine, tobacco) which increase needs for micronutrients and add to the toxic burden.
- Genetically modified foods – most genetic modification is aimed at making crops pesticide resistant, so more sprays can be applied, or sprays that are intrinsically more toxic to pests are applied, but in either case that puts a detox burden on the human liver.

There is no one-size-fits-all diet. The starting point for all healthy people is to observe all the above rules. However, for patients who come to see me with some health problem, the diet may have to be further honed according to other factors. The common starting points I use are as follows for otherwise healthy people with no symptoms and no disease:

- No added sugar or refined carbohydrates. However, the occasional carbohydrate feast will not upset a healthy gut. Indeed, primitive man would have had such during the autumn to fatten up prior to winter.
- No dairy products, except butter, ideally ghee. It is milk *protein* which should be avoided as it contains growth promoters and may be carcinogenic.
- Initially avoid addictions, such as alcohol and caffeine. (Dry cider in my case!) Then use judiciously.
- No fruit juices which are rich in addictive sugars, especially fructose. High-sugar fruits should be avoided. Berries are usually fine; however, even strawberries are being so cultivated that they are becoming too sweet.
- Eat fermented foods such as kefir and sauerkraut.

- Avoid chemical additives. Eat as organically as possible. Eat foods in season, locally grown for freshness.

My advice on meals is:

- Breakfast like an emperor, lunch like a king, sup like a pauper.
- Only eat at mealtimes, with a knife and fork. Eat slowly and chew. Snacking means the stomach never has a chance to become fully acid. We need an acid stomach to prevent upper fermenting gut and to protect against infection.
- One day a week of fasting or major calorie restriction – for example, 500 kcals at breakfast and none for the rest of the day. This is highly protective against metabolic syndrome (and weight gain) and is of course evolutionarily correct. Primitive man did not eat three regular meals a day.

As you start to switch to the Paleo-ketogenic diet you may feel worse initially. This is to be expected for the following reasons:

- Hypoglycaemia symptoms – This is the commonest reason for worsening and may take weeks to settle. It is difficult for the body to switch from fuel delivery by carbohydrates to fuel delivery by fats.
- Caffeine withdrawal – Again, this is common and usually results in a headache which clears in four days.
- Food allergy withdrawal symptoms – Coming off foods for which there is an intolerance may cause many different symptoms. Some people report feeling 'flu like. Typically this lasts four days, but symptoms like eczema, arthritis, allergic muscles and fatigue can take weeks to clear. One patient with enlarged prostate took four months to clear his symptoms.
- Herxheimer reactions – These are allergic reactions to gut flora detritus as fermenting microbes die off.
- Possibly, detox reactions as the body gains the energy and reserves to offload some toxins. Weight loss results in the same since many chemicals are mobilised.
- Perhaps to allow the gut flora to change. Carbohydrate-based diets result in high levels of prevotella; fat- and protein-based diets result in high levels of bacteroides.

I advise patients to go into the diet gently, perhaps over several weeks. Start with establishing a good cooked breakfast, using nuts and seeds for snacks, then establish supper and finally lunch. The diet needs to evolve slowly so that it becomes sustainable for life. The occasional indiscretion is acceptable; it is the everyday insults which damage.

A useful clue to knowing you are on a low-carbohydrate diet has to do with the mouth. Teeth will feel glassy smooth, as if they have been polished at the dentist. They will be free from plaque (bacteria colonies).

B. Micronutrients:
multivitamins, minerals and essential fatty acids

Westerners all need to take supplementary micronutrients for life for the reasons given previously. My standard package (what I call MMM) is:

- Multivitamins – containing at least 25 mg of B1, B2, B3, B5, B6 vitamins, 1 mg of folic acid, 1 mg of B12, vitamin A 2,000 IU, vitamin E 50 mg and vitamin K 0.2 mg.
- Multi-minerals – The following doses of elemental weight are per 2 stone (12.5 kg) of body weight: calcium 60 mg, magnesium 70 mg, potassium 40 mg, zinc 6 mg, iron 3 mg, boron 2 mg, iodine 0.3 mg, copper 0.2 mg, manganese 0.2 mg, molybdenum 40 mcg, selenium 40 mcg, chromium 40 mcg. These doses should be taken up to a maximum dose for a 10 stone (62.5 kg) person – that is, up to five times the amounts listed above. Use 1 gram of mix per litre of water; this can also be used to make hot drinks. I do not include sodium chloride (salt) because this is contained in so many foods. If absent, then sea salt should be used, approximately 1 gram per 2 stone of body weight per day and capped at approximately 2 grams per day.
- Vitamin D – at least 2,000 IU daily, but up to 10,000 IU daily.
- Hemp oil – one dessertspoonful, together with two capsules of fish oil.
- Vitamin C – at least 2 grams, possibly up to 10 grams at night.

These doses assume that nothing comes from the diet. However, as the Paleo-ketogenic diet is adopted and when sun bathing is possible, these doses can be reduced.

C. Sleep

One cannot create energy and function without doing some damage. All living creatures, right down to bacteria, require rest, when systems are shut down to allow healing and repair. We call this sleep. Without a good night's sleep on a regular basis all other interventions are to no avail.

First, get the physical essentials in place:

- A regular pre-bedtime routine – Your 'alarm' should go off at 9 pm, at which point you drop all activity and move into your bedtime routine.
- A regular bed time – 9.30 pm at the latest to take proper advantage of hormones that support growth and repair. Earlier in winter, later in summer.
- Your day needs the right balance of mental and physical activity.
- Do not tolerate a bed fellow who snores – you need different rooms!
- A high-fat, low-carbohydrate snack just before bedtime (such as nuts, seeds) helps prevent nocturnal hypoglycaemia, which often manifests with vivid dreams or sweating or waking in the night. However, some people find any food disturbs sleep and they sleep best if they do not eat after 6 pm.
- Perhaps restrict fluids in the evening if your night is disturbed by the need to pee.
- No stimulants, such as caffeine, or adrenaline-inducing TV, arguments, phone calls, family matters or whatever immediately before bed time! Caffeine has a long half-life – none after 4 pm.
- Dark room – the slightest chink of light landing on your skin will disturb your own production of melatonin (the body's natural sleep hormone); have thick curtains or blackouts to keep the bedroom dark; this is particularly important for children. Do not switch the light on or clock-watch should you wake.
- A source of fresh, preferably cool, air.
- A warm, comfortable bed – We have been brainwashed into believing a hard bed is good for us and so many people end up with sleepless nights on an uncomfortable bed. It is the shape of the bed that is important. It should be shaped to fit you approximately and then very soft to distribute your weight evenly and avoid pressure points.
- If your sleep is disturbed by heat and sweating then this is likely to be a symptom of low blood sugar. Menopausal sweats are worsened by hypoglycaemia.
- If sleep is disturbed by pain, try to find the cause. In the short term, one must just take whatever pain killers are necessary to control this. However, many pain killers are also anti-inflammatory and will suppress the immune system. The immune system is responsible for healing and repair and this should take place at night.
- If you wake in the night with symptoms such as asthma, chest pain, shortness of breath or indigestion, then this may point to food allergy being the problem, with these withdrawal symptoms occurring during the small hours.

Then get the brain off to sleep:

- Learn a 'sleep dream' to train the subconscious to switch on the sleep button.
- Learn to recognise the sleep wave – one comes every 90 minutes; be in bed ready to ride it with the sleep dream.
- If you do wake in the night, do not switch the light on or get up and potter round the house or you will have no chance of dropping off to sleep. Use your sleep dream again.

Getting the physical things in place is the easy bit. The hard bit is getting your brain off to sleep. Throughout life, the brain makes a million new connections every second. This means it has a fantastic ability to learn new things. Getting off to sleep is all about developing a conditioned reflex. The best example of this is Pavlov's dogs. Pavlov was a Russian physiologist who showed that when dogs eat food, they produce saliva. He then 'conditioned' them by ringing a bell whilst they ate food. After two weeks of conditioning, he could make them produce saliva simply by ringing a bell. This of course is a completely useless conditioned response, but it shows us the brain can be trained to do anything.

Applying this to the insomniac, firstly one has to get into a mind set (sleep dream) which does not involve the immediate past or immediate future. That is to say, if you are thinking about reality then there is no chance of getting off to sleep.

There is a time for many words, and there is also a time for sleep.

HOMER, *The Odyssey*, eighth century BC

Then you use a hypnotic (see opposite) which will get you off to sleep. You apply the two together for a period of 'conditioning'. This may be a few days or a few weeks. The brain then learns that when it gets into that particular mindset, it will go off to sleep. Use of the hypnotic medication should become unnecessary. However, things can break down during times of stress and a few days of medication may be required to reinforce the conditioned response. But it is vital to use the correct 'mindset' every time the medication is used, or the conditioning will weaken.

I do not pretend this is easy, but to allow one's mind to wander into reality when one is trying to sleep must be considered a complete self-indulgence. Treat your brain like a naughty child. It must simply not be allowed to free-wheel.

Find a sleep dream that suits you

If you think about real events, then there is no chance of dropping off to sleep. You have to displace these thoughts with a sleep dream. It could be a childhood dream, or recalling details of a journey or walk, or whatever. It is actually a sort of self-hypnosis. What you are trying to do is to 'talk' to your subconscious. This can only be done with images, not with the spoken language since your subconscious deals with emotions and feelings. I dream that I am a hibernating bear, snuggled down in my comfortable den with one daughter in one arm and the other in the other. Outside the wind is howling and the snow coming down and I am sinking deeper and deeper down . . .

Learning a sleep dream is a bit like riding a bicycle – it looks impossible at a distance but with a bit of practice becomes easy. Your brain will try to convince you that a sleep dream is not working, but that is just because the brain likes to free-wheel – especially if you are naturally hyper-vigilant!

Initially use medication to reinforce the sleep dream

I instinctively do not like prescribing drugs. However, in cases of ingrained insomnia, I do use them for sleep, in order to establish the above conditioning and to restore a normal pattern of sleep, after which it should be possible be tail off or keep them for occasional use. Indeed, viruses can cause neurological damage (for example, polio) and this could involve damage to the sleep centre. Some people are constitutionally hard-wired for hyper-vigilance and may need medication for life to allow them to sleep.

When it comes to sleep medication, I am always asked about addiction. My experience is that this is rare, especially if drugs are used as above to develop a conditioned reflex or to treat pathologically awful sleep. One has to distinguish between addiction and dependence. We are all dependent on food, but that does not mean we are addicted to it. We are all dependent on a good night's sleep for good health and may therefore become dependent on something to achieve that. This does not inevitably lead to addiction. Addiction is a condition of taking a drug excessively and being unable to cease doing so without other adverse effects. Stopping your hypnotic may result in a poor night's sleep but little more than that. This is not addiction, but dependence.

Medication for sleep

I recommend:

- **Melatonin** (see page 98) 3 mg (one tablet) 1–3 tablets at night. Some people just need 1 mg. I suspect melatonin deficiency is what I call an 'acquired metabolic dyslexia' (see page 190) – as we age we may all benefit from additional melatonin at night. It is additionally a good antioxidant.

- **Nytol** (diphenhydramine) 50 mg. This is a sedating antihistamine available over the counter. The dose is ½–2 tablets at night. This is long acting – don't take it in the middle of the night or you will wake feeling hung-over.
- **Valerian root** 400 mg (1–4 capsules) at night. This is a herbal preparation which is shorter acting and can be taken in the middle of the night.
- **Kava kava.** I used to find this very useful but unfortunately it has now been banned in the UK.

If there is no improvement with a combination of the above, or if there are intolerable side effects, then I would go on to a prescribed drug. I usually start with one of the sedating antidepressants such as:

- **Amitriptyline** 10–25 mg. I would start with 5 mg initially. (Most CFS/ME patients are made worse and feel hungover with 'normal doses'.)
- **Trimipramine** 10–30 mg at night – a longer-acting version of the above.

Some insomniacs need prescription tranquillisers, such as temazepam 10–20 mg (short acting), zopiclone 3.75–7.5 mg (medium acting) or clonazepam 0.5–2 mg (long acting).

It is vital to combine the above prescriptions with a good sleep dream and all the above interventions. Do not let the medication work without, otherwise tachyphylaxis (a decrease in drug response) will result, and the medication will become ineffective.

D. Exercise – the right sort to give benefit

> If we could give every individual the right amount of nourishment and exercise, not too little and not too much, we would have found the safest way to health.
>
> HIPPOCRATES, the father of medicine (460–370 BC)

Humans, along with all other mammals, evolved living physically active lives. This usually meant long hours of sustained activity, but there would be occasions when maximal energy output was needed – for example, to fight an enemy or bring down prey. Internal metabolism is fully geared to physical activity and without this we cannot be fully well.

We need exercise as we need food and water: in just the right amount. Too much risks injury and muscle damage; too little and we degenerate. To maintain optimal fitness, we need steady sustained exercise combined with outbursts of extreme energy. Just as with food, the type of exercise and the amount is critical. After research and practical application, Dr Doug McGuff and John Little produced their book *Body by Science – a research-based program for strength training, body building and complete fitness in 12 minutes a week*. Thanks to their work, we can now see how to exercise most efficiently (see page 80). We do not want to do so much that we wear out our body (this is what happens with so many athletes – most runners are carrying injuries) but when we do exercise it must be effective to improve cardiovascular fitness. What is so interesting about McGuff and Little's approach is how well this correlates with what we already know about mitochondria, blood sugar control and fats.

Their approach makes perfect evolutionary sense. I do not see badgers and foxes trotting round my hill every morning to get fit! Most of the time wild animals are in hiding or feeding quietly. Once a week there will be a predator–prey interaction – the predator must run for his life to get his breakfast; the prey must run for his life to avoid being breakfast; in so doing, both parties will achieve maximal lactic acid burn. This is all that is required to get fit and stay fit.

The underlying principles

We are taught that there are two types of fitness – namely, muscle power and cardiovascular fitness. Not so. What drives cardiovascular fitness is muscle strength. When muscle strength is used to its full capacity, it creates a powerful stimulus to the energy supply mechanism. This includes mitochondrial function and heart function. The heart pumps blood to send fuel and oxygen round the body, where is it picked up by mitochondria in the cells which convert that to ATP, the currency of energy in the body. This means that if muscle strength is correctly developed, this automatically translates into cardiovascular fitness and increased numbers of mitochondria. More mitochondria means better cardiovascular fitness. Most importantly, McGuff has an excellent research base to show that only 12 minutes a week is needed to achieve this.

What this means is that cardiovascular fitness is the same thing as mitochondrial fitness. Getting fit is actually about supplying the right stimulus to mitochondria to get them geared up to speed and to increase their numbers. If the mitochondria can supply the energy, then the muscle can work at a high level and maintain that.

How does exercise impact on mitochondria?

The body has to gear its energy use very carefully in order that energy is used most efficiently. To achieve this there are three types of muscle fibre. On the one hand we have 'slow-twitch', on the other 'fast-twitch', with intermediate fibres between the two.

Slow-twitch fibres – These are used when power demands are low. This makes them very efficient; they use small amounts of energy and give good endurance so that we can use them for a long time. They are rather weak fibres but are slow to fatigue and quick to recover. These are the fibres we use for pottering about when we do not need much power.

Intermediate-twitch fibres – If we work a bit harder we start to recruit intermediate twitch fibres.

Fast-twitch fibres – These are employed when power demands are high. They occupy much more space and give us big muscles; they require a lot of energy to cope with high power demands, fatigue very quickly and take a long time to recover once fatigued.

What happens when you start to use muscles – recruitment

The brain controls whether slow-twitch or fast-twitch fibres are used. It wants energy to be used in the most efficient way, with quick recovery. So initially it employs the slow-twitch fibres. If the power demands are low, these fibres stay in use. Energy supplied from the blood stream is sufficient. This is what we do when we potter. Trained athletes can run very efficiently just using slow-twitch fibres. These people are thin with smallish muscles. They make the best long-distance runners.

If the power demand increases, the brain also starts to recruit the fast-twitch fibres. This requires much more energy to cope with the power demand, and energy stores within the muscle – that is, glycogen stores – are quickly used up. Athletes with highly developed fast-twitch muscles are the sprinters and weight lifters – they have large powerful muscles. I believe these people are much healthier than the long-distance runners because they are not wearing out their bodies.

Strong fast-twitch muscle fibres afford huge metabolic benefits

This is because:

- During power exercise, glycogen in the muscles is used up. This is excellent news. Sugar is one of the fuels of the engine – highly effective but highly dangerous. When blood sugar levels rise after a meal, the best sponge for mopping it up is muscle and liver glycogen. Normally this is depleted by exercise, but without exercise, glycogen remains saturated, blood sugar levels spike and the hypoglycaemia roller-coaster is triggered.

- If glycogen stores are never depleted, then sugar gets shunted into fat instead. This means any carbohydrate consumed results in fat (obesity) and the formation of the 'bad' cholesterol LDL. High levels of LDL are symptomatic of the wrong sort of exercise and therefore indicate poor mitochondrial function and so poor cardiovascular fitness. High LDL is symptomatic of metabolic syndrome.
- Depleting glycogen activates the hormone-sensitive enzyme lipase so that fats are mobilised from body stores and made available for energy supply. This is very helpful for the dieters who get stuck.
- If sugar in the blood stream following a meal cannot be taken up because glycogen stores are full, then this excess sugar sticks on to other things creating 'advanced glycation end products' or AGEs (see page 191) – they literally accelerate the normal ageing process. One such example is 'glycosylated haemoglobin', which is measured to assess blood sugar control in diabetics.

Remember:
Good fast-twitch fibres = good mitochondrial function = good cardiovascular fitness

The right sort of exercise (see below) creates a demand for energy. Initially this energy comes from Krebs citric acid (KCA) cycle, which is anaerobic (without oxygen) and provides pyruvate for oxidative phosphorylation. In this scheme, KCA provides two molecules of ATP and happens very fast. Oxidative phosphorylation is slower to get going but provides 36 molecules of ATP. Athletes call this delay 'getting a second wind'.

If energy demands increase further (see below) we use both aerobic and anaerobic metabolism and the latter generates lactic acid. This gives us our lactic acid burn, renders exercise uncomfortable and makes us want to stop.

But the important point about lactic acid is that it provides a powerful stimulus to our energy supply system – that means, mitochondria and heart function, or cardiovascular fitness, in other words. More mitochondria means bigger muscles. (Each heart cell has 2,000–3,000 mitochondria, occupying most of the cell.) Big muscles mean lots of mitochondria, mean good cardiovascular fitness. It really is a case of 'no pain, no gain', but the good news is that with correct exercise the pain is only short lived.

So what sort of exercise?

To increase muscle bulk and improve cardiovascular fitness one needs to do the right sort of exercise:

- The exercise has to be very slow but powerful – this prevents damage to muscles and joints.
- It must be sufficiently powerful so that initially the slow-twitch fibres are used, but towards the end of the exercise all the fast-twitch fibres are being used. If the exercise is not demanding enough, then only the slow-twitch fibres will be used – so no gain!
- The window of time to exercise a group of muscles needs to be 45–90 seconds.
- At the end of this window, the muscles being worked must be burning with lactic acid and weak – that is to say, the exercise cannot be sustained any longer. This means your fast-twitch fibres have all been fully employed and exhausted. This provides the maximum stimulus for improved energy supply (and therefore cardiovascular fitness) and enlarging muscles. Since over half of muscle weight is mitochondria, big muscles mean more mitochondria. What makes muscles fatigue is not lack of muscle filaments, but inability to supply energy to them. When men show off their muscles, actually they are showing off their mitochondria.

The slow-twitch fibres will recover quickly, so after a few minutes you will be able to function normally, but you will not be able to repeat the power exercise you have just done. If you can, then you have not done enough! This mild muscle damage is a powerful stimulus to create more mitochondria.

- After exercising a group of muscles, they must be rested for a few days (that is, stay within slow-twitch capabilities); this allows time for healing and repair to upgrade mitochondria, make more mitochondria and better functioning fast-twitch muscle fibres.
- There is no gain to be had from repeating these exercises more often than once every few days – the heart and mitochondria only need one good kick to upgrade their performance. Indeed, repeat exercises are likely to be counter-productive by causing too much tissue damage.

Remember, wild animals are all super fit, but most of the time they are pottering about gently or hiding. It is only occasionally that either the predator has to put in a powerful burst of activity to catch his prey or the latter has to do likewise to escape. This is how Nature keeps them fit!

What are the actual exercises?

There are many options, all with enthusiastic advocates. But time is always at a premium and anything you do must be incorporated into busy life in a way that is sustainable in the long term. To increase and maintain fitness I do two things – I walk my dog daily up a steep hill as fast as I can – only walking – so my legs ache and I puff and pant. Twice a week I do 20 press-ups. All else, such as riding, walking or gardening is just for fun.

Intensive exercise

When fit, trained athletes (usually distance runners) suddenly drop dead, it is likely this is due to acute magnesium deficiency. Deficiency in the general population is common, but for every mile run, about 10 mg of magnesium is lost in sweat and urine. One needs calcium to contract heart muscle and magnesium to relax it – so deficiency may cause the heart to stop in systole. By post mortem, minerals have leaked out of cells and the diagnosis is missed. For intensive exercise it is important to rehydrate with an electrolyte mix that contains multi-minerals. After sweating I recommend 1 gram of my standard multi-mineral mix with 2 grams of salt in 1 litre of water to rehydrate.

E. Sunshine and light

> Where there is sunshine, the doctor starves.
>
> FLEMISH PROVERB

Sunshine on the skin is highly desirable for at least three reasons.

To make vitamin D from UV light

Western cultures have become almost phobic about any exposure of unprotected skin to sunshine. Indeed, the US Environmental Protection Agency advised that ultraviolet light, and therefore sunlight, is so dangerous that we should 'protect ourselves against ultraviolet light whenever we can see our shadow'. That advice is just nuts! As the Maori proverb goes: 'Turn your face to the sun and the shadows fall behind you.'

The best source of vitamin D is sunshine – not so much that the skin burns, but enough to tan. One hour of whole-body exposure to Mediterranean sunshine can produce 10,000 to 20,000 IU of vitamin D. We need at least 2,000 IU daily, and probably more for optimal health. No studies have shown any toxicity in doses up to 10,000 IU daily. Further excellent information can be found at www.vitamindcouncil.org.

I use high-dose vitamin D routinely in the treatment of multiple sclerosis, any condition associated with inflammation (allergy, infection, autoimmunity), osteroporosis and arthritis. My CFS/ME patients are nearly always deficient. Note that the normal blood levels for NHS labs are set very low at 30–60 ng/ml. I like to see levels at 75–200 ng/ml.

Whilst sunshine exposure is a risk for basal and squamous cell cancer, these are relatively benign, easily treated and rarely kill. At the first sign of sun damage to skin I recommend Curaderm – extract of eggplant. It is highly effective in treating solar keratosis, early basal cell carcinoma (rodent ulcers) and early squamous cell carcinomas. If there is no sign of remission after eight weeks of use, then consultant opinion is necessary.

There is increasing evidence that sunshine is not a risk factor for aggressive melanoma. If it were then this tumour would have the same distribution as other skin tumours. It does not.

Do not use sun tan lotions. There is evidence to suggest that they increase cancer risk directly or, because they give a false sense of security, then they increase cancer risk indirectly through complacency. Once there is a risk of burning, head for the shade or cover up.

To make us happy

Absence of full-spectrum light results in SAD (seasonal affective disorder). This is no fun but evolutionarily desirable – it helps us conserve energy through long, cold winters because we do not want to do things – boring, but with survival advantage. Sunshine is addictive – indeed, one measure of addiction is how much money we are prepared to spend on such. Holidays in hot climates are expensive but still highly desirable.

To receive heat in the form of far infrared (FIR)

Such free heat means we do not have to generate so much heat from our own mitochondria. This too has survival benefits as an energy conservation method. Indeed, the mitochondria of native Africans run slower than Caucasians', and much slower than Inuit Indians'. The latter have a high metabolic rate and are excellent at fat burning, which is essential to deal with the cold. They need abundant food to fuel this demand. By contrast, native Africans run their mitochondria slow, and this makes them much more susceptible to metabolic syndrome and all its complications. They are metabolically highly efficient.

We use this form of heat in FIR saunas to detoxify chemicals. However, I suspect this is just one of many possible benefits of FIR about which we have much more to learn. The heat from muscular activity radiates as infrared. This warming reduces friction in connective tissue to reduce stiffness.

F. Reduce the chemical burden

We live in an increasingly polluted world containing an increasing number of chemicals which are toxic to our genes, to our brains, to our internal metabolism and to our immune system. These 'nasty' toxic chemicals contribute to our ever-increasing incidence of cancer and birth defects and our declining fertility, due to lifetime exposure, and also make us more susceptible to chronic fatigue syndrome.

It is impossible to completely avoid every 'nasty' chemical. I have yet to do a fat biopsy or measure toxic metals in urine following DMSA challenge (see page 197) and find a normal result. We live in equilibrium with our environment and the best we can do is keep the total toxic load as low as reasonably possible. Anything which can be done to reduce the toxic chemical load will be helpful in allowing our bodies to recover.

Dr Paula Baillie Hamilton in her book *The Detox Diet: Eliminate Chemical Calories and Restore Your Body's Natural Slimming System* explains how chemicals in foods and the air interfere with internal metabolism to make us fat and lethargic. Indeed, she points out that farm animals are deliberately fed hormones, antibiotics and pesticides to make them fat and lethargic, and therefore they do not have to eat so much in order to put on weight (cheap meat). Effectively we are treating our farm animals to produce a metabolic syndrome. Many chemicals are persistent and concentrate up through the food chain – it is very likely that if Westernised humans were a farm animal they would be declared too toxic to eat.

Reduce your chemical exposure

It is impossible to avoid the 'nasty' chemicals altogether, but we can do a fair amount to limit our exposure.

FOODS

- Eat the best quality food you can find.
- Choose foods grown as naturally as possible; if organic food is available, go for it.
- Eat foods that are as unprocessed as possible; most foods in tins or packages have preservatives or have been irradiated.
- Eat foods which have not been plastic wrapped; the plasticiser gets into food.
- Avoid foods wrapped in aluminium foil, or in aluminium cans.

- Eat fresh foods; if they have to be stored, deep freezing is probably the least harmful.

WATER

A clean water supply is essential. The water companies are only interested in bacterial counts – they will not measure pesticide levels, heavy metals, hormone residues, volatile organic compounds or fluoride in your tap water. Water should at least be filtered to remove heavy metals and pesticide residues. More recently, chloramine has been used instead of chlorine – this may be cheaper for the water companies but it is less effective at killing microbes than chlorine, more toxic, and not removed by simple water filters. Bottled water in plastic containers may be contaminated with phthalates, so glass bottles are worth the trouble and expense.

AIR

- If you can smell it, it can make you ill – the obvious offenders are cigarette smoke, air fresheners, sprays, perfumes and cleaning agents, but there are a host of other chemicals in everyday use. Some used-car sales companies now spray their cars to make them smell like brand new cars as this improves the chances of a sale!
- If you can't smell it, it could make you ill! Such is the case with carbon monoxide poisoning. It may present with CFS. Have a CO monitor in your kitchen or anywhere where you have a gas- or coal- burning appliance and always have good ventilation.
- New paints and carpets (especially rubber-backed, stuck down) give out toxic fumes for months after; use water-based paints wherever possible.
- Soft furniture and furnishings are routinely treated with the fire retardants poly-brominated biphenyls. These are known carcinogens; I routinely find them in fat biopsies.
- Pesticides – dog and cat flea treatments, fly repellents, house fumigations and timber treatments all contain toxic pesticides which may persist for months if not years. I have many patients with CFS/ME following such chemical exposures.
- Gas central heating and gas cookers can make some people ill.

COSMETICS

- **Deodorants:** Most deodorants contain aluminium which, when applied to warm sweaty areas, is readily absorbed. Aluminium is toxic and has a recognised association with Alzheimer's disease. It is an immune adjuvant with the potential to switch on allergy and autoimmunity.

- **Hair dyes:** I often see hair dyes in toxicity tests, such as DNA adducts (page 198) and translocator protein studies (page 229). Hair dressers have an increased risk of cancer.
- **Perfumes:** Perfumes and 'smellies' can be a real problem, especially where there is multiple-chemical sensitivity. Look at the work of Campaign for Safe Cosmetics www.safecosmetics.org.

GARDEN AND AGRICULTURAL CHEMICALS

Gulf War syndrome, sheep dip 'flu and aerotoxic syndrome are examples of severe life-threatening conditions caused by organophosphate pesticides and other such chemicals. These chemicals are extremely toxic. Children with leukaemia are twice as likely as those without to have lawn chemicals applied at home. Many country dwellers are subject to spray drift. I have some patients who have to leave their homes during the spraying seasons to avoid acute ill health.

SOCIAL AND PRESCRIPTION DRUGS

These may substantially increase the overall toxic load so that, in addition to being toxic in their own right, they increase the toxicity of other chemical burdens. This is because they all use the same detoxification pathways which then become overloaded. I suspect this is the mechanism by which many of my CFS/ME patients are markedly intolerant of many prescription drugs. **Head lice treatments** contain toxic pesticides and should not be used at all. Lice can be controlled with wet combing or electric 'zappers'.

OUTDOOR AIR POLLUTION

I believe the late Dr Dick van Steen did more for the health of the nation than any other doctor through his campaigning work against polluting industry. He demonstrated increased risks of cancer, heart disease, respiratory disease and birth defects close to and downwind of such. Many industries discharge pollutants directly into the local air, water and soil. The worst offenders are power stations that burn toxic waste, the manufacturing industry and the chemical industry. Power stations often burn SLFs (secondary liquid fuels). This is where the spent, dirty oil drained from your car during its service may end up. Busy roads create traffic fumes. Toxic chemicals are dumped at waste sites where they pollute ground water, soil and air. You need local knowledge to identify these issues. Ask specifically about:

- Heavy metals – arsenic, cadmium, nickel, copper, lead, aluminium, etc.
- Radioactive waste.

- Pesticide residues – organochlorines and dioxins, organophosphates, pyrethroids, etc.
- Small particulate matter (down to PM 1 micrometre and less – don't settle for PM 10 size: PM 10 can be seen as smoke; PM 1 or less is invisible).
- Volatile organic compounds (VOCs) – solvents, benzene compounds
- Polluting gases (SOx, NOx, COx – sulphur, nitrogen and carbon compounds).

We are now seeing epidemics of lung cancer in people who have never smoked. I suspect this is due to the above outdoor air pollution.

GOOD NUTRITION

This is highly protective against toxic stress, and is a further reason to take nutritional supplements. One example of this came out of the research into thalidomide. This drug prescribed to women in pregnancy as a 'pregnancy-safe hypnotic' (sleeping pill) caused serious birth defects if the women took it during early pregnancy. But not all babies were affected. This drug was tested in rats – no offspring were abnormal. This was a mystery to researchers, until someone had the bright idea of putting the rats onto nutritionally depleted diets. Then the baby rats developed the foetal abnormality of phocomelia ('flipper limbs'). It was a combination of toxic stress (the drug) and nutritional deficiency which caused the problem to become apparent.

G. Sufficient physical, mental and financial security to satisfy our universal need to love and care, and be loved and cared for

It is beyond the scope of this book to discuss the psychological and spiritual imperatives that we must fulfil for optimal physical and psychological health and I am no expert. I am deeply grateful for a loving carefree childhood with a Mum who was a brilliant cook. This love flowed further to my two gorgeous daughters, Ruth and Claire, but as they became more independent my affections embraced my pets – horses and more recently my lovely puppy, Nancy. Pets are far more emotionally intelligent and sensitive than humans! I think it is essential for anyone living alone, or in an emotionally lacking relationship, to have a loving pet.

My horizons are constantly changing. When my girls were little, my hobby was watching them have fun. Most recently I want my house, which is too big for one, to become the Marigold Hotel for horse and dog lovers. Humans evolved to live in tribes, certainly not to live alone and probably not just within a single family. A complex social life is vital to good mental health.

Simply identifying the above needs is often helpful to patients. Knowing what they need, they then come up with innovative solutions.

H. Avoid infections

Acute infections clearly cause short-term misery, but I am more concerned by their potential to switch on CFS/ME, allergies, autoimmunity and cancer. Even arterial disease may have an infectious component – it is clearly driven by inflammation. Many cancers we know are infection driven, such as cervical cancer (human papilloma virus, HPV), stomach cancer (*Helicobacter pylori*), Kaposi's sarcoma (HIV infection), Burkitt's lymphoma (Epstein-Barr virus), hepatoma (hepatitis B), lung cancer (tuberculosis), and so on. We also know many cases of autoimmunity are infection driven. I suspect that the upper fermenting gut will eventually prove to be the major risk factor for oesophageal, stomach and colon cancer.

Avoiding infection is an important part of long-term good health.

How to avoid infection

- Keep warm – cold kills. When the mistral wind blows in France, death rates increase.
- Drink clean water and eat clean food.
- Take care with sexual partners – passionate love is a form of insanity that makes us do insane things and take insane risks!
- Avoid insect bites with the potential for blood-to-blood transmission of pathogens. We are seeing epidemics of Lyme disease from biting insects.
- Treat breaches of the skin thoroughly – keep clean and wrap up. All animal bites get infected. I have seen infections of heart valves and inter-vertebral discs arising from such.
- Eat a low-carb diet and especially avoid sugar and fruit sugar – these are the substrates that microbes love to ferment. New cases of diabetes may be picked up because of recurrent thrush, fungal toenails or staphylococcal skin infections.
- Dental hygiene – the commonest chronic infection is *Streptococcus mutans*, which causes dental decay, with gum disease resulting eventually. Dental decay is a marker symptom of many other diseases, including the clinical

picture of metabolic syndrome and of course upper fermenting gut. Avoid sugar, brush teeth regularly and perhaps use herbal antiseptic mouth-washes, such as neem.

- Identify and treat hypochlorhydria – an acid stomach is a major line of defence against infection. Microbes that are inhaled stick to the mucous lining of the airways and are coughed up and swallowed – so most end up in the stomach. This should be an acid bath to sterilise the upper gut. This is therefore particularly a problem where there is hypochlorhydria (insufficient acidity). Hypochlorhydrics are at increased risk of food poisoning and recurrent infections.
- Do not graze – this never allows the stomach time to become fully acidic between meals.
- Take probiotics regularly – these are of proven benefit in, for example, avoiding traveller's diarrhoea.
- Take micronutrients as per the Basic Package – these are essential for normal immune function.
- Vitamin C – this is toxic to bacteria, viruses and fungi (and, incidentally, cancer cells). It is harmless to normal cells. It is a fabulous defence against infection. Taken by mouth it is poorly absorbed, but that helps protect against infection via the gut.

I advocate taking a dose of vitamin C last thing at night on an empty stomach. The idea is to reduce microbial numbers in the upper gut by killing the millions of microbes in the upper gut (those fermenting or ingested) but not sufficient to kill the billions of microbes in the lower gut. Too much vitamin C will do the latter and result in diarrhoea. Take vitamin C to doses just below. Linus Pauling, winner of two Nobel Prizes, championed vitamin C and took 14 grams daily. He lived to 93.

DO NOT BE OBSESSED WITH HYGIENE AND CHEMICAL DISINFECTANTS

Such measures may be counter-productive. You can never sterilise a surface – microbes will always be present. The immune system needs normal exposure to everyday microbes for correct programming. Mothers are usually fastidious with first-born babies, less so with the rest; first-born children are more likely to suffer from allergy.

A child who is protected from all controversial ideas is as vulnerable as a child who is protected from every germ. The infection, when it comes

– and it will come – may overwhelm the system, be it the immune system or the belief system.

JANE SMILEY (1949–)

SYMPTOMS OF ACUTE INFECTION SHOULD NOT BE SUPPRESSED WITH DRUGS

Symptoms arise to make us do the things we need to do to reduce numbers of microbes (cough, wheeze, sneeze, etc), or to conserve energy and resources for fighting infection efficiently (rest, sleep). Only too often my CFS/ME patients tell me they had an infection and continued to work by dint of taking paracetamol, caffeine, antihistamine or pseudoephedrine, then turned to addictions to cope with the stress, so allowing their virus to get topside. This is short-term gain, long-term pain.

2. The bolt-on extras

We do not have all the tools to treat all the problems, but the body is fabulous at healing itself. We only have to get the package 51 per cent right and the body will do the rest. Only 49 per cent right and one is on the slippery downhill slope. Many tools multitask. For example, ATP is the energy molecule and also a neurotransmitter; high-dose vitamin B12 may be used to improve mitochondrial function, for detoxing via the methylation cycle (see page 106), as an antioxidant and for its anti-inflammatory properties by damping down the pro-inflammatory fire of the NO/ON/OO cycle (see page 220).

I. Tools to treat acute infection

All of the above! And more:

- **Feed a cold, starve a fever:** The gut and liver are greatly demanding of energy – empty the gut by fasting and energy is freed up for the immune system to burn hot and run a fever.
- **Hydrate with water, salt and minerals:** Where there is fluid loss through sweating, diarrhoea or vomiting, rehydrate. My recipe is 1 litre of water with 2 grams of salt (a teaspoon is 5 grams, so half a teaspoon) and 1 gram of multi-mineral mix (as in the Basic Package micronutrients – see page 67), drunk ad lib.

- **Rest:** Again, this allows the immune system the essential resources it needs to deal with infection. Do not exercise. Some athletes claim they can run off an acute infection – this may be because that generates heat which kills microbes, but it is a high-risk policy.
- **Encourage a fever:** Keep warm.
- **Do not use symptom-suppressing medication** for all the reasons given in this chapter.
- **Vitamin C,** taken in sub-diarrhoeal doses at the first sign of a cough or cold, will often prevent the illness from progressing. High-dose vitamin C should be used in any acute infection. Many doctors use high-dose intravenous vitamin C in the treatment of infection and cancer, with good results reported. Up to 50 grams (50,000 mg) daily are used intravenously; this demonstrates how safe this vitamin is.
- **High-dose probiotics** – I suggest kefir, 1 to 3 cupfuls daily.
- **Use antiviral herbal preparations,** such as colloidal silver 20 ppm (one dessertspoonful rinsed round mouth, gargle and swallow, three to four times daily), echinacea (25 drops held in mouth and then swallowed three to four times daily) or propolis (600 mg three times daily). It is really a case of trying as many things as you can until you find a combination that suits you.
- **Zinc drops or lozenges:** Take 10 mg four times daily into the mouth to kill microbes. Zinc is the commonest mineral deficiency that results in poor immunity. It is directly toxic to microbes. I use an infection spray which contains vitamin C, zinc and colloidal silver in DMSO (derived from tree bark) for topical use on skin and mucous membranes.
- **Antibiotics, antifungals and antivirals** all have their place; I would not like to practise medicine without them. They should be used to reduce numbers of microbes when patient defences are compromised. They will prove much more effective when the above interventions are also in place.

II. Tools to treat poor energy delivery
a. Poor mitochondrial function

As described before (see page 32), mitochondria are the power houses of all cells – the 'ultra-structures' in the cells where glucose is converted to ATP, which is the body's energy currency. Broadly speaking, mitochondria go slow either because they lack substrate (glucose and oxygen) to work efficiently, or because they are blocked by toxic stress. (There are other reasons.) Dr Stephen Sinatra's excellent book *The Sinatra Solution* identifies the common biochemical bottlenecks that result in poor function – his ideas find good biochemical support in the tests of mitochondrial function that I do in my CFS/ME patients. The ageing process is determined by mitochondria, so as we age perhaps we should all be taking additional supplements to support our mitochondria. Dr John McLaren-Howard, Dr Norman Booth and I published a paper (the third in a series) in January 2013 which showed that those CFS patients taking the package of supplements I advocate to support mitochondrial function and remove sources of toxic stress (chemicals from the outside world or products of the upper fermenting gut), improve biochemically and that this improvement is paralleled by clinical improvement. This paper can be seen at www.ijcem.com/files/IJCEM1207003.pdf.

The package that I use is as follows:

- Coenzyme Q10 250–500 mg daily (the oil of the engine). It is virtually impossible to overdose with co-Q10.
- Acetyl L-carnitine 1–2 grams daily (the fuel pipe that delivers the acetate fuel into mitochondria).
- Vitamin B3 (niacinamide) 1,500 mg slow release (an essential step between the Krebs citric acid cycle and the process of oxidative phosphorylation).
- Magnesium 400 mg orally, perhaps injections. (I think of magnesium as the spark plug of the engine.)
- D-ribose 5–15 grams – the raw material to make new ATP, the energy molecule.
- Vitamin B12 1–2 mg daily, ideally by injection.

VITAMIN B12

Vitamin B12 is very poorly absorbed and to be used as a therapeutic tool is best given by injection. It is very safe – it has no toxicity; the only way you could kill yourself with vitamin B12 would be to drown in the stuff! I teach my patients to self-inject; this is very easy to do. I would start with 1 mg subcutaneously daily, in the morning (it may cause insomnia if used at night). The technique is identical to that used by diabetics self-injecting with insulin.

A few micrograms a day prevent pernicious anaemia and it is on this basis that 'normal ranges' have been set. However, many need much higher doses for optimal biochemical functioning. Many do not feel well until blood levels are above 2,000 pg/ml – a 'normal' blood level is no reason not to try B12 injections. The frequency of dosing depends on clinical factors – that is, how the patient feels, not blood tests. The most bioavailable form is methylcobalamin. I use up to 5 mg (5,000 mcg) daily by injection to treat:

- Physical fatigue – racehorses are regularly injected with B12 because they then run faster.
- Mental fatigue – I was intrigued to hear that chess grandmasters inject themselves daily with B12 to improve mental performance.
- Dementia – in my view, if doctors were serious about preventing dementia then everyone over the age of 60 would receive a monthly B12 injection.
- Depression – in theory, one should be careful in manic depression because mania can develop on high-dose injections; however, I have never seen this happen.
- Almost any neurological disorder, especially multiple sclerosis and peripheral neuropathy.
- Where tests show poor antioxidant status.
- Where tests show poor conversion of ADP to ATP.
- Where tests show poor methylation.
- Anyone over the age of 60, for a combination of the above reasons.
- If I can't think of anything else to try!

MAGNESIUM FOR ENERGY PRODUCTION

Magnesium is at the heart of energy production. Indeed, as I have said, I think of magnesium as the spark plug of the engine. There is a particular vicious cycle with magnesium: 40 per cent of all energy generated by mitochondria is needed to power the ion pumps that kick calcium out of cells and drag magnesium in, ditto sodium versus potassium. Magnesium is needed by mitochondria; the mitochondira are within cells; if they go slow they cannot generate the power to pull in the magnesium they need for energy generation.

I suspect this explains why magnesium injections are so superior to oral supplements. They spike levels of magnesium in the blood which reduces the concentration gradient across cell membranes and hence also reduces the work load of the ion pumps. Suddenly magnesium can get into mitochondria, so they can function.

I think of magnesium injections as kick-starting the mitochondrial engine. I suggest 0.5 ml of 50 per cent magnesium sulphate (1 gram in 2 ml) subcutaneously daily. The technique is the same as for injecting B12. This delivers 25 mg of elemental magnesium. It astonishes me that such a small amount can be so effective when the recommended daily amount is 350 mg!

In addition to its effects on mitochondria, magnesium is essential to relax muscles and nerves. Calcium excites and fires up muscles and nerves; magnesium does the opposite. Magnesium has been dubbed 'Nature's tranquilliser'.

These combined effects mean that taking magnesium intravenously is very helpful for a wide range of conditions. By injection, it is of proven benefit in the treatment of angina, migraine, acute myocardial infarction, acute stroke (when caused by thrombosis), peripheral vascular disease, malignant hypertension, eclampsia, the muscle spasm of the airways in asthma and the spasm of bowel muscle. In my work as an NHS GP, I used intravenous magnesium in emergency medicine more than all other forms of treatments put together. I learned this technique from Dr Sam Browne who published in the *Journal of Nutritional and Environmental Medicine* in 1994.[9] I additionally use intravenous bolus injections in my CFS/ME patients who have corrected all that can be corrected metabolically but whose 'engines' seem to need kick-starting with a larger dose of magnesium. The Browne paper suggests up to 6 ml of 50 per cent magnesium sulphate can be delivered in an intravenos injection given slowly over two minutes. I use a fine orange needle to inject because this preserves the vein – one patient has received, I estimate, over 100 intravenous magnesium boluses through the same vein; she died recently aged 101.

VITAMIN B3

When I measure blood levels in fatigue syndromes, almost invariably they are deficient in B3, even in people who are already taking a standard B complex. Many people need 1,500 mg slow-release to correct levels, some twice this dose. Vitamin B3 is essential to make nicotinamide adenosine diphosphate (NAD) – the intermediary between the Krebs citric acid cycle and oxidative phosphorylation (essential for energy production). So any condition requiring energy may benefit from high dose B3. It is of proven benefit in chronic fatigue syndrome, diabetes, in many mental disorders with psychosis (see the work of Dr Abram Hoffer[10]), arthritis (see the work of Dr William Kaufman[11]) and some degenerative neurological diseases, such as Alzheimer's.

BLOCKING OF MITOCHONDRIA

This may result from exogenous toxins (see detox regimes, page 105), endogenous toxins (see fermenting gut, page 201) or because of poor membrane quality (for which, consume high-dose hemp oil with quality fish or shell fish oils).

b. Thyroid function – the accelerator pedal of our car

UK citizens are not subject to 'Best Practice' with respect to prescribing thyroid hormones. All relate to the prescribing of thyroid hormone for underactive thyroid glands (hypothyroidism).

THE THRESHOLD FOR THYROID-STIMULATING
HORMONE IS SET TOO HIGH

When levels of thyroid hormones in the blood start to fall, the pituitary gland increases its output of thyroid-stimulating hormone (TSH), which kicks the thyroid into life and increases output of thyroid hormones. If the thyroid gland starts to fail, this is reflected by levels of TSH rising. The question is, at what point should the prescription of thyroid hormones begin?

The normal range for TSH in the UK varies enormously from one laboratory to another. This means in some locations a thyroid prescription would not be given until the TSH rose above 5.0 mlU/l. As a result of research, the normal range for TSH in America has now been reduced so that anybody with a TSH above 3.0 is prescribed thyroid hormones. This research has shown that people with a TSH above 3.0 are at increased risk of arterial disease. What is completely illogical is that in the UK the target TSH level for patients on thyroid replacement therapy is often stated as being less than 2 or even less than 1.5. This is a ridiculous anachronism given that prescription is not recommended until levels exceed, say, 5.0 mlU/l. We should reduce the threshold for prescribing thyroid hormones to a TSH above 3.0 mlU/l, or possibly above 2.5 mlU/l. This applies especially to pregnancy when requirements increase by 50 per cent. The level of thyroid hormones in pregnancy is critical for foetal development.

POPULATION REFERENCE RANGE
VERSUS INDIVIDUAL NORMAL RANGE

The population reference range and the individual normal range are not the same. We differ as individuals in our biochemistry as we differ in our structure and brains. This biochemical variation should be taken into account when it comes to prescribing thyroid hormones. The population normal range for free T4 (thyroxine) is 12–22 pmol/l. A patient, therefore, with blood levels of 12.1 may be told he/she is normal because the level is within the population reference range. But actually that person's personal normal range may be high. They may feel much better running a high T4 of say 22 – that is, nearly twice as much but still within the population reference range. This is the commonest form of hypothyroidism in CFS/ME where there is a general suppression of the hypothalamic-pituitary-adrenal axis (see page 208).

POOR CONVERSION OF INACTIVE T4 TO ACTIVE T3

There are two thyroid hormones – T4 (thyroxine) and T3. T4 must be converted to the active form (T3) for the metabolism to run normally. Poor conversion can sometimes be predicted from bloods tests where T4 is high and

T3 is low. This is not always the case, however – levels of T3 fluctuate through the day and so the blood tests may not always be an accurate measure.

THYROID HORMONE RECEPTOR RESISTANCE

Some people only feel well using pure T3 as a supplement, not T4; at present we do not have biochemical tests to predict who these people are.

STARTING TREATMENT WITH THYROID HORMONES

The starting dose of thyroid hormones depends on the degree of abnormality of the blood tests, and the size of, and the robustness of, the patient. Small, unwell patients should be started on just 12.5 mcg thyroxine daily, then increase their dose in 12.5 mcg increments every two weeks until they get to 50 mcg daily, at which point one should recheck the biochemistry. At all times the patient should remain euthyroid – that is, show no symptoms of too much thyroid hormone. These symptoms include tremor, anxiety, insomnia, palpitations and other such; monitoring needs to be done by a doctor. Most people need 75–200 mcgms of T4 or its equivalent. The exception to this is where there is thyroid hormone receptor resistance where higher doses may be needed to see a clinical response.

There are currently no tests available to diagnose thyroid hormone receptor resistance. This is a similar scenario to type II diabetes, where there is insulin resistance and yet measuring insulin levels is unhelpful.

Equivalent doses: thyroxine 75 mcg =
one grain of natural thyroid = 60 mg of natural thyroid =
15 mcg of pure T3 (l-thyronine)

If T3 is part of the treatment, because it is short acting and has a marked circadian rhythm, the dose must be split so half the daily dose is taken ideally 90 minutes before wakening (tricky – this needs an alarm to wake sufficiently to take a pill but not enough to prevent further sleep), a quarter at midday and a quarter late afternoon. Further tweaking may be necessary to fine-tune the timing. If T3 is being used, then I recommend Paul Robinson's book *Recovering with T3* which goes into great clinical detail. Also see www.thyroiduk.org.uk/tuk/index.html.

MAINTAIN TREATMENT

Once up to the dose where there is clinical improvement, wait four weeks for blood levels of thyroid hormones to stabilise and then re-check free T4, free

T3 and TSH levels, re-assess things clinically and continue to adjust according to the above parameters. It may take several months to see the full clinical benefits. Once stable, bloods can be re-checked every year, sooner if problems arise, then every two to three years.

If pure thyroxine is used, aim for blood levels of free T4 in the top half of reference range, with a TSH of about 1.0. Fine-tune the dose further, according to clinical factors.

If natural thyroid is used, expect to see 'highish' levels of free T3 and 'lowish' levels of free T4. This is because the proportion of T3 to T4 in these preparations is high.

If pure T3 is used, expect to see free T4 be very low, often less than 1 pmol/l. That does not matter – it is T3 which is the active hormone. If T3 is being used because of thyroid hormone receptor resistance then blood levels are unhelpful. They may be very high.

PREGNANCY

Requirements for thyroid hormones increase 50 per cent during pregnancy. The neurodevelopment of the baby is exquisitely sensitive to thyroid hormones so it is essential to re-check bloods every three months and again after delivery.

c. Adrenal function – the gear box

Where there is complete failure of the adrenal gland, most commonly due to autoimmunity, treatment is life-saving and must be overseen by a consultant endocrinologist. However, in clinical practice this is rare. What I most often see is adrenal fatigue, or partial adrenal failure. This can be diagnosed with an adrenal stress test. This is done on four saliva samples taken through the day. Arguably, saliva tests are better than blood tests because the latter can be coloured by 'protein binding'. Saliva tests are a measure of the free available hormone.

INTERPRETATION OF THE ADRENAL STRESS TEST
FOR DHEA AND CORTISOL

Levels of DHEA and cortisol vary according to the level of stress the individual is experiencing and for how long that stress has been applied. Increasing cortisol production is the normal response to short-term stress and is highly desirable, so long as the stress is removed and the adrenal glands can recover. Ongoing, unremitting stress means the adrenal gland and the whole body are in a constant state of alert, do not get time to recover and eventually pack up. So, there are several stages of adrenal function gradually leading to failure:

Normal levels of cortisol and DHEA, normal circadian rhythm – Normal result.

Raised cortisol, normal DHEA – This indicates a normal, short-term response to stress, of which the commonest cause is falling blood sugar levels, but it can be any stressor.

Raised cortisol and raised DHEA – The adrenal gland is functioning normally but the patient is chronically stressed. So long as the stress is removed, the adrenal gland will recover completely.

High levels of cortisol, low levels of DHEA – This is the first sign of partial adrenal failure and the first abnormal adrenal response to chronic stress. The patient needs a long break from whatever that chronic stress may be. DHEA can be supplemented to make the patient feel better, but it must be part of a package of recovery to address causes of stress, without which long-term worsening can be expected. Depending on the result, I prescribe between 10 and 25 mg sublingually to take in the morning. Furthermore, I suspect that low DHEA is an 'acquired metabolic dyslexia' (see page 190) – levels fall with age, and physiological supplementation (that is, 10–20 mg daily) may be helpful to mitigate the effects of ageing. Increasingly, I am swapping over to pregnenolone 50–100 mg daily; metabolically this is immediately downstream of cholesterol and the mother hormone of all steroid hormones. In the future I hope this will simplify regimes.

Cortisol levels low, DHEA levels low – The adrenals are so exhausted they can't make cortisol or DHEA. By this time, patients are usually severely fatigued and this hormonal picture is typical of CFS/ME. Often there is loss of diurnal rhythm with no morning spike. In addition to attention to stressors upstream and DHEA or pregnenolone supplements, as above, I prescribe hydrocortisone cream 1 per cent. A normal adrenal gland should produce 20–25 mg of hydrocortisone over 24 hours. Depending on the level, I prescribe 1–2 ml of cream (10–20 mg) applied to the skin daily. This dose is physiological so there are no side effects and no suppression of the hypothalamic-pituitary-adrenal axis. Remember, low morning cortisol may be symptomatic of hypothyroidism.

In addition to absolute levels, this test may indicate poor diurnal rhythm of hormones. If levels of DHEA are low in the morning, this may indicate low melatonin at night. In this event, I prescribe 3–9 mg of melatonin per night, especially if sleep is disturbed.

d. Circadian rhythms – timing is vital

Early to bed, early to rise, makes a man healthy, wealthy and wise.

BENJAMIN FRANKLIN (1706–1790)

RE-ESTABLISHING THE CIRCADIAN RHYTHM

Modern Western lifestyles destroy our natural circadian rhythm because of light (inhibiting melatonin production at night), noise (disturbing sleep), diet (hypoglycaemia and adrenalin disturbing sleep), drugs of addiction (withdrawal symptoms), caffeine and other such. Interventions that help include:

- Bright light, ideally sunshine, by day
- Complete darkness at night
- Peace and quiet at night
- High-fat breakfast for energy delivery – diet should be Paleo-ketogenic (see page 223)
- Physical and mental exercise during the day
- Bed by 9 pm, asleep by 9.30 pm – the best quality sleep occurs before midnight
- Melatonin 1–9 mg at night, perhaps other medications – see sleep section (page 72)
- Take thyroid hormones in the morning on waking (T3 sooner) – levels of TSH peak at midnight, T4 peaks at 4 am and T3 at 5 am
- Take cortisol and DHEA (or pregnenolone) on wakening
- Perhaps use caffeine in the day to fire up – but none after 2 pm
- Perhaps B12 injections in the morning to fire up
- Other things as I (and the patient!) learn more

III. Tools to treat inflammatory conditions

Reduce the pro-inflammatory load

Correct poor energy delivery mechanisms – When these go slow, more free radicals are produced.

Allergen avoidance: foods, food additives, biological inhalants, chemicals and microbes – Just as with infection, it is a number's game. Allergy is all about total load and if this can be reduced below a critical threshold then tolerance develops.

Improve foods – The Paleo-ketogenic diet is an excellent start and may be all that is necessary to reduce the total load. Where there are obvious and known reactions to foods, avoid them. If this becomes impossible, then rotation diets are helpful; the idea here is to eat a food once every four days so one allergic insult does not come on top of another. Quick and efficient digestion of foods means large, antigenically interesting molecules are rapidly broken down to minimise the potential for sensitisation, so improving gut function is important. Apply the tools to treat the upper fermenting gut (see page 201).

Avoid biological inhalants – Generally speaking, these are large, water-soluble molecules. Simple masks filter out much of the allergens – if I am grooming my horse or moving hay I just tie a tea towel over my nose and mouth, otherwise I risk a session of sneezing and wheezing. In the event of any reaction, a shower and change of clothing is very helpful. (House dust mites thrive in soft furnishing and soft toys.)

Address chemical sensitivity – Many sufferers are exquisitely sensitive; I know those who react to washing powders on clothes on the neighbours' washing line, perfume on passers-by and discharges from polluting industry. Sometimes avoidance is impossible. Air filters are helpful. Sufferers may be reacting to POPs contained within their own fat, so reducing the endogenous load of POPs using tools for detoxification (see page 105) is helpful.

Microbes – The main source is microbes from the upper fermenting gut, so use the tools to treat such (see page 102).

Tools to help damp down the pro-inflammatory biochemical fire of the NO/ON/OO cycle

The following can help reduce the pro-inflammatory effect of the NO/ON/OO cycle (see page 220):

Correct poor antioxidant status – Simply taking the Basic Package of nutritional supplements of vitamins and minerals will go a long way towards correcting poor antioxidant status. However, I routinely measure levels of antioxidants, and deficiencies are common. I would use in response to the following deficiencies:

- Superoxide dismutase – Copper 1 mg at breakfast, manganese 3 mg midday, zinc 30 mg at night; these timings reflect the time of day these nutrients are best absorbed.
- Glutathione peroxidase – Glutathione 250–500 mg, selenium 200–500 mcg at night.

- Coenzyme Q10 – 250–500 mg daily
- Other important antioxidants, such as vitamins A, C, D and E, are part of the Basic Package. There are many natural antioxidants within our diet which are additionally helpful. These are found in vegetables, nuts, seeds and berries.

Vitamin D evolved in response to sunshine on skin as an anti-inflammatory to protect the skin from pro-oxidant stress from ultraviolet light. It diffuses through the body where today it has generalised anti-inflammatory actions. It is protective against infection and improves muscular strength. It also protects against allergy, autoimmunity, metabolic syndrome, osteoporosis and cancer. The incidences of all these conditions increase the further away from the Equator you live. It is important to measure blood levels in anyone with any of these conditions since absorption can be variable. I like to see levels between 75 and 200 nmol/l. To achieve this requires up to 10,000 IU daily.

Vitamin B12 by mouth and by injection – This provides instant antioxidant cover and protection whilst the other antioxidants are being corrected by supplements. See page 91 for details and dose.

Alkalinisation – The use of bicarbonates and carbonates has long been recognised as a way to switch off allergy reactions, especially to foods. I suggest magnesium carbonate 500–2,000 mg last thing at night, or at least away from mealtimes. We need a window of time (at least 90 minutes after food) to achieve an acid stomach to allow normal gut function. Magnesium carbonate may be additionally useful if acid supplements are being used to treat hypochlorhydria.

Low-dose naltrexone (LDN) – Naltrexone is an opiate blocker used in high doses, such as 50 mg, to block the effect of opiates. LDN is used in tiny doses, such as 1–4 mg at night. The idea is to slightly block opioid receptors, which results in an increase in endogenous production of endorphins. Endorphins are natural anti-inflammatories. This property gives LDN wide clinical application, from the treatment of cancer to autoimmunity and neurodegenerative disorders. See www.lowdosenaltrexone.org for detailed information.

Exercise, music, singing, love and laughter – All are addictive because they increase endorphins with anti-inflammatory actions arising downstream. Some addictions are useful!

Desensitising techniques to turn off allergies – enzyme potentiated desensitisation (EPD) and neutralisation

The mainstay of treating allergy is avoidance. Problems arise when allergens are multiple or unavoidable. The technique I use is EPD (see page 199) but comparative studies of EPD and neutralisation (see page 219) give similar long-term outcomes. Both treatments are fabulously safe because the concentrations of antigens in the mixes are extremely low. Both have been proven to work in placebo-controlled double-blind trials. Both techniques can be used to desensitise to foods, biological antigens (pollen, dusts, animal dander, etc), microbes and chemicals.

EPD seems to work by reprogramming the immune system to respond appropriately. The idea here is that the bone marrow constantly sends out new white cells which mature and are programmed by the status quo. EPD reprogrammes these naive cells to respond appropriately to the antigens present in the injection. It may take several injections before sufficient cells are correctly programmed and allergy is switched off.

ADVANTAGES OF EPD

- All the common antigens are represented in the vaccine so I do not have to know all the antigens to which a patient is reacting for the treatment to be effective.
- The injection is easy to administer and takes just a few seconds . . .
- But it may take some months to see improvements.
- I can use EPD as a one-man band. This makes it relatively inexpensive. In my NHS General Practice I used to keep EPD in the surgery fridge and use it regularly for many conditions associated with allergy; most surgeries would see someone have an injection!
- Sometimes I use EPD in my CFS patients because I do not know what else to try! Often I am pleasantly surprised by the results, suggesting that allergy is a major and often unrecognised player in the cause of fatigue.

ADVANTAGES OF NEUTRALISATION

- A result can be seen immediately, but . . .
- Each antigen has to be identified and desensitised individually – this may take up to an hour, so treatment is time-consuming and expensive.
- The neutralisation points can change, which means the patient often has to return for further testing.

ORAL IMMUNOTHERAPY

The idea of oral immunotherapy is to start with tiny doses, build these doses up slowly, and as a result, over time, the immune system will develop tolerance to that particular substance. This technique was used in the NHS during the 1970s to treat pollen allergies. At that time, it was given by injection, starting off with tiny doses, and then the dose would be increased every week until after about 10 weeks tolerance to grass pollen was achieved in the majority of patients. Unfortunately, this type of low-dose immunotherapy was banned because some authorities started to use multiple allergens. This use of multiple allergens meant that, in order to prevent immediate reactions, the allergen mixes were put in an oil-soluble medium so that the antigens would be released slowly. The effect of this change in administration technique was that, if a patient was going to suffer a serious reaction, then this serious reaction happened at home because of the delayed release effect. This in turn meant that patients were suffering serious reactions where basic resuscitation assistance was not available. As a result some patients died, leading to a ban of this kind of low-dose immunotherapy. The baby was thrown out with the bath water!

Recently, a new study has been published demonstrating how anaphylactic reaction to peanut can be 'switched off' by administering tiny doses of peanut by mouth and then by gradually increasing the dose of peanut slowly over time.

I do not see why this idea could not be extended to all foods and with this in mind I have prepared some food mixes made up of 100 different foods. One would then start off with a very low dose, say 1–2 mg a day (that is, the same dose as the peanut anaphylactic study). If this was not tolerated, then one would reduce the dose. If it was tolerated, then one would gradually increase the dose. This recent idea I have included in this book because not only is it biologically plausible but there is huge potential to help many people for whom there is no other easy and affordable therapy. However, I am on a steep learning curve.

HOMEOPATHY

I am no expert but I have seen many patients who are greatly helped by homeopathy. I suspect one possible mechanism of action is that it re-programmes the immune system to respond appropriately. Homeopathic doctors tell me that their remedies work much better when the Basic Package is also applied.

IV. Tools to improve gut function

Reduce bacteria and yeast in the mouth – Use a low- or zero-carb, ketogenic diet. The fermenting gut may start with bacteria and yeast in the mouth. These are inevitably swallowed. I find neem toothpaste and neem mouth wash helpful; neem is toxic to the microbe *Streptococcus mutans* which causes dental decay.

Low/zero-carb ketogenic diet – Eat a diet of low-fermentable substrate. The only foods that do not ferment are fats and oils. How do I know this? I can leave a lump of lard in my fridge for weeks and it does not ferment (it may oxidise and go rancid, eventually, but that is not fermenting). I can leave a bottle of olive oil in my pantry for months and it does not go off. Proteins as in meat, fish and vegetables, may be fermented by microbes which are also fermenting carbohydrates. So the essence of the diet is low, or even no, carbohydrate. Less commonly, there is upper fermenting gut by anaerobic bacteria, which will ferment vegetable fibre, but the commonest starting point for therapy is a zero-carb ketogenic diet.

Improve digestion – Ensure good digestion of food:

Hypochlorhydria (low stomach acid) is often found in association with the fermenting gut; take acid supplements, such as betaine hydro-chloride 325 mg 1–5 capsules, or ascorbic acid 3 grams, or the juice of a whole lemon, with meals. Some people use cider vinegar, but this may be a problem if yeast allergy coexists. Taking exogenous acids will acidify the body generally, so if necessary, mitigate the effect with alkali, such as magnesium carbonate 500–2,000 mg at night.

Pancreatic enzymes are often helpful; there are many preparations on the market.

Bile salts – 1–3 grams of mixed bile salts should be taken with meals.

Probiotics physically displace and compete for substrate. They also help modify the immune system in the gut – 90 per cent of the immune system is gut associated. Probiotics will not colonise the gut (none survive it), but they will do much good en route. Eat fermented foods, such as sauerkraut and kefir (which can be grown on soya, coconut or rice milks). Kefir is inexpensive – one sachet will last a lifetime as cultures can be grown from previous.

Transdermal supplements – Don't feed microbes with B vitamins and minerals; microbes in the gut are as hungry for raw materials as human cells. I often recommend transdermal supplements, which can be applied to the skin with a carrier molecule (DMSO) in order to bypass the gut.

Vitamin C – This is to kill off the fermenting microbes. Vitamin C is toxic to all microbes; the key point is the dose. I suggest a single large dose at night and adjust according to bowel tolerance (that is, take until diarrhoea just threatens, then reduce the dose slightly). The idea is to take sufficient vitamin C to kill the millions of microbes in the upper gut but not sufficient to kill the billions of microbes in the lower gut. Vitamin C is poorly absorbed, but this is ideal for the purposes of treating the upper fermenting gut.

Antimicrobials – It may be that the above is all that is necessary to treat a fermenting gut, but some patients need specific antimicrobials in addition. Tests are helpful and a comprehensive digestive stool analysis gives us an idea of which microbes and which antimicrobials are necessary. However, what I do know is that the battle against the fermenting gut is not a battle; it is a war. Given the right substrate, microbes can double their numbers every 20 minutes. I suspect one can never reduce their numbers to zero. The best one can do is get numbers so low that they no longer cause problems for reasons of either infection or allergy. I think of this as siege warfare – the principles are the same! (Once ahead of the game be careful not to let regimes slip too much.) Think of your gut as your garden – you can keep the numbers of weeds down but never get rid of them. The main triggers are sugar, fruits and refined carbohydrates – the occasional dose may bump numbers up from a few hundred to a few thousand, which is no problem, but with regular sugar consumption, soon one has millions of microbes happily fermenting again.

Antifungals:

    Pure nystatin powder is a pleasure to use because it is effective and cannot be absorbed, meaning it has no toxicity. The dose is titrated up according to clinical factors. Expect to get die off, or Herxheimer-like reactions – this is thought to be an allergic reaction to dead yeast antigen. Such reactions may be very severe. See www.drmyhill.co.uk/wiki/Nystatin_-_how_to_take_it for details of dosing regimens. (Thank you, Dr John Mansfield, for this regime.)

    Itraconazole 100 mg od (once daily) and fluconazole 100 mg od are both excellent antifungals. However, there is the potential for liver toxicity so liver function tests need checking monthly. Having said that, I rarely see problems because good nutrition is highly protective against toxic stress and I advise all my patients to take micronutrients.

Herbals – There are many such with proven antifungal/antibacterial actions. Combinations may be more effective because resistant strains are less likely to emerge. Try to include these in the diet: artemesia, garlic, oregano, berberis, uva ursi, golden seal, plant tannins, mastic gum, grape fruit seed extract and others. I am on a steep learning curve here! This is where herbal medicine may be very useful. I do use prescription antibiotics, but there is much less collective experience than with antifungals. The problem with antibiotics is that there are so many strains of bacteria with the potential to ferment that knocking one back may leave a vacuum in which another may flourish.

Worms – Humans evolved with worms. Evidence suggests that the immunoglobulin IgE exists to deal with worm burdens in the gut. I see worms as occupational therapists for IgE! Africans with high IgE carry a lower worm burden and this gives them an evolutionary edge. In modern Western societies we do not have significant worm burdens so perhaps IgE makes trouble in other areas, resulting in atopic allergy. Hookworms have been used with good results in inflammatory bowel disease. It may be they could be helpful in atopic diseases such as eczema, asthma, urticaria and anaphylaxis.

Faecal bacteriotherapy – The most important probiotics, which make up 90 per cent of the gut flora, are the obligate anaerobes, such as bacteroides which ferment vegetable fibre in the large bowel. These do not survive oxygen and so there is no probiotic on the market which contains bacteroides. The idea of faecal bacteriotherapy is to replenish the gut with these friendly bacteria using a fresh specimen from a healthy donor. This treatment has been pioneered by Dr Thomas Borody (centrefordigestive diseases.com). We now have a clinic in the UK that offers this treatment (www.taymount.com). This treatment is of proven benefit in inflammatory bowel disease and *Clostridium difficile* infections. It is also used in the veterinary world to treat animals with a range of gut symptoms. There is now also evidence that this therapy is beneficial in CFS. I have no experience of using faecal bacteriotherapy but it is a logical and safe treatment. This is another steep learning curve for me.

Bacteriophages – This is a treatment for the future. The idea here is that bacteria have their own predators in the form of viruses. These are specialised to attack bacteria and are not toxic to human cells. Whilst Western countries developed antibiotics, Eastern Europe developed bacteriophages. It may be that many of the benefits of faecal bacteriotherapy arise because friendly phages are also being introduced into the gut; indeed, much of the normal gut flora are phages.

V. Tools to detoxify

a. General approach

Remove the polluting source – There is no point doing detox regimes without also addressing the issue of where the toxins are coming from. The upper fermenting gut is a major source of toxic stress. I would not advocate chelation therapy for toxic metals such as mercury until the source of the toxin, such as dental amalgam, has been removed.

Ensure good energy delivery – The business of detoxing is greedy for energy and resources. Most occurs in the liver which, at rest, consumes 27 per cent of total body energy production. This is more than the brain and heart combined.

Ensure good micronutrient status – Most toxins are rendered water soluble, first by oxidation by cytochrome P450 enzymes and then by tacking on a group such as glucuronide, glutathione, sulphate , amino acid or other such. So, for example, if I measure levels of glutathione in the body, in someone who is not taking supplements, almost invariably there is a deficiency. Glutathione is in great demand for detoxing and also for glutathione peroxidise, which is a vital antioxidant.

There are many other ways by which the body can detoxify: many fat-soluble chemicals can be got rid of in the bile (but are then, unfortunately, reabsorbed in the gut); other toxins can be eliminated in faeces; some toxins are exhaled; some sweated out of the body, or boiled off – as I call it – from the subcutaneous fat onto the lipid layer of the skin, which can then be washed off.

Treatment depends on the toxin involved, but certain steps should be applied in every case. The following enhance the body's ability to detox:

- Apply all the Basic Package interventions: Paleo-ketogenic diet, micronutrient supplements, sleep and exercise.
- Avoid constipation and thirst.
- If applicable, and it often is, treat the fermenting gut.
- Avoid identifiable sources of exogenous toxic stress.
- Correct nutritional deficiencies – Possibly measure levels of minerals, such as magnesium, zinc and selenium; minerals are essential cofactors of, confer special properties to, and allow enzymes to work.
- Glutathione 250–500 mg daily is very helpful. Glutathione is almost invariably deficient when I measure it and corrects reliably well with supplements. There are other sulphur-containing compounds which may be equally helpful, such as methionine 250–500 mg daily, N-acetyl cysteine, alpha lipoic acid and many others.

b. Correct the methylation cycle

Simply taking the Basic Package of nutritional supplements of vitamins and minerals (see page 72) will go a long way towards correcting poor methylation. But there is a particular vicious cycle here – vitamins B12 and folic acid, essential parts of the methylation cycle, need to be methylated before they can be of use. Sometimes they must be given in the methylated form to be effective. The following regime helps:

- Methylcobalamin 1 mg sublingually (but ideally by injection) daily
- Methyltetrahydrofolate 800 mcg (ActiFolate) daily
- Pyridoxal-5-phosphate 50 mg twice daily
- Glutathione 250 mg daily
- Phosphatidyl serine 100 mg twice daily

c. Specific regimes

GETTING RID OF TOXIC METALS

Trace minerals – Toxic metals bio-accumulate because of deficiencies of essential trace elements (often a metal). The idea here is that if an element such as zinc is deficient (and this is common), the body will grab something that looks similar. This means toxic metals such as lead or cadmium get incorporated into the body instead, with dire results. So treatment is to give a larger than usual dose of trace elements to displace the toxic one. This is combined with a sulphur-containing protein, such as glutathione or methionine, to which the toxic metal sticks and the conjugate produced is dumped in the urine.

Glutathione 250–500 mg or methionine 250–500 mg – So a typical regime to counteract poisoning with nickel, lead or cadmium (divalent cations) would be: zinc 30–50 mg at night, with methionine or glutathione 250–500 mg daily. A typical regime to counteract aluminium, mercury and arsenic poisoning (trivalent cations) would be selenium 500 mcg at night, with methionine or glutathione 250–500 mg daily.

Vitamin C, 4 grams daily – If tolerated, the best form of vitamin C is ascorbic acid and the slight acidity will render the urine acidic, which helps to strip out toxic metals.

High-dose iodine, 12.5 mg once daily (e.g. Iodoral one tablet) – Iodine sticks to toxic metals to make a soluble iodide which can be excreted.

DMSA – Strips out many toxic metals remarkably well. We know this simply by measuring toxic metals in urine following a dose of DMSA. Indeed, this is an excellent test for toxic metals. The only problem is that some people do not tolerate DMSA very well, in which case we have to rely on the above interventions. If tolerated, DMSA is the most reliable way of stripping out mercury, lead, arsenic, cadmium, aluminium and others. I would use DMSA 15mg/kg of body weight once a week. DMSA also strips out essential trace-elements so take no mineral supplements on these days. The rest of the week, rescue with physiological doses of essential trace elements in addition to the above regimes. Duration of treatment depends on the degree of toxicity, but usually lasts at least 16 weeks. There is no evidence that DMSA gets into the brain, but reducing levels in the body creates a gradient conducive to toxic metals coming out of the brain.

Mobilising toxic metals can make the patient worse – Perhaps because of toxic and allergic reactions to the mobilised metal, mobilising toxic metals can make things worse. With my 'sensitive flowers' I start with small doses and adjust according to response. Some people just do not tolerate DMSA at all.

Whatever regime is used, re-test toxic metals in urine – This gives two points on the graph so an educated guess can be made at how much more treatment, if any, is required. If the levels do not come down as expected, then there are two possible reasons. Either there is ongoing contamination from an unidentified source, or there is redistribution of toxic metals – sometimes it is like peeling off layers of an onion as heavy metals seem to come out in quantum leaps. One just has to continue detox therapy until a downward trend is seen. Every milligram of DMSA pulls out a load of toxic metals.

Clays such as kaolin and bentonite – I try this for people intolerant of DMSA. I do not have enough data to be sure that it is effective, but there is every reason to suppose that this would work. Again, it would be expected to pull out essential trace elements so I suggest 5 grams three times daily, twice a week, in a similar pulsed way to DMSA. On clay days, don't take trace minerals (except perhaps trans-dermally, because these would not enter the gut) and then rescue with physiological doses of trace elements as done with DMSA.

GETTING RID OF PESTICIDES AND VOLATILE ORGANIC COMPOUNDS THROUGH HEATING REGIMES

The source of heat does not matter too much – exercise, hot baths, sauna and sunshine should all be effective. However, many patients, especially my severe CFS/ME patients, are intolerant of heat. This is where **far-infrared (FIR) sauna-ing** is helpful. FIR heat penetrates several centimetres into the skin and subcutaneous tissue to mobilise chemicals without initially increasing core temperature. This way the heat is much better tolerated. Indeed, it is likely that FIR has other benefits over and above simple heating; perhaps this is part of the reason why we love to lie in sunshine – sunshine addiction seems very common! It also seems to give us well-being and energy.

The idea behind FIR sauna-ing is that toxic chemicals that have been dumped by the body in fat, including subcutaneous fat, are shaken up and boiled off through the skin where they dissolve on the lipid layer on the skin surface. Showering these chemicals off is as important as sauna-ing – otherwise they are simply reabsorbed. It is not necessary to sweat for FIR sauna-ing to be effective – indeed, most chemicals come out in the first 5–10 minutes of sauna-ing – so little and often gets the best results. Should there be excessive sweating, then rehydration should include minerals and salt (1 gram of multi-minerals and 2 grams of salt in 1 litre of water). Sweat is serum-less cells and large molecules – all minerals will be present in sweat.

Roughly speaking, 50 FIR saunas will halve the load – chemicals come out exponentially so a further 50 saunas will reduce the total load to 25 per cent of total and so on. One can never get rid of every last molecule. One ends up in a state of equilibrium with the environment – and of course all environments are polluted.

I have done fat biopsies and DNA adducts and gene studies on 27 patients before and after FIR saunas. Levels of pesticides and VOCs come down reliably well. It may be there are other techniques that work just as well, such as exercise (but not for my CFS/ME patients), traditional saunas (again, not tolerated by CFS/ME patients) and hot Epsom salt baths (500 grams of Epsom salts in 15 gallons of water; soak for 30 minutes – indeed, Epsom salt baths may be additionally effective because, as the chemicals come out, magnesium and sulphate are absorbed, so providing valuable detox raw materials). These techniques all should, in theory, work just as well. However, I do not yet have data to support them.

Some people are made ill even by FIR sauna. I suspect this partly results from chemicals being mobilised into the blood stream where they cause an acute poisoning. FIR sauna-ing does not get rid of toxic metals.

d. Phospholipid exchange
FATS, OILS AND ESSENTIAL FATTY ACIDS (EFAS)
Fats, oils and essential fatty acids (EFAs) are the essential building blocks from which cell membranes are made. Nearly all biochemical processes take place on cell membranes. These hold enzymes in just the right 3D configuration to allow biochemistry to proceed efficiently. Modern Western diets and lifestyles are inherently toxic and the pollutants involved bioaccumulate in fat and membranes, with major potential to disrupt normal enzyme function. Simply consuming large amounts of clean organic fats and oils helps to displace these toxic oils. Dr Patricia Kane uses high doses of these clean oils intravenously and claims remarkable successes in a range of neurological disorders.

In the UK, the Burghwood Clinic offers phospholipid exchange – see www .burghwoodclinic.co.uk.

I recommend high-dose organic oils orally containing omega-6 and omega-3 EFAs in the proportion four to one for purposes of detoxification. Hemp oil is naturally very close to this ratio.

WATER

I do not advocate drinking excessive water as a method of detoxing. One can drink pure water but one cannot pee pure water, so friendly minerals are washed out and lost. Some of the worst-nourished people I see are those who believe it is healthy to drink several litres of water a day. An adequate intake for men is roughly 3 litres (about 13 cups) of total beverages a day and for women 2.2 litres (about 9 cups) of total beverages a day, assuming no excessive sweating. Water should be taken with multi-minerals and salt (if not already in the diet).

Conclusion

There are clearly other methods of detoxification that are effective, but because the above interventions work reliably well, I stick with these methods. Importantly, I have a good evidence base to support their use.

VI. Tools to treat mechanical problems: structure, friction and wear and tear
Structural problems

The human body is intrinsically unstable and needs powerful, coordinated muscles to allow it to function. Look at yourself in the mirror – most people are not symmetrical. Furthermore, they tend to tip forwards. If you are not sure, then ask an athlete, a personal trainer, a physiotherapist or whoever to teach you correct posture. Learn to exercise correctly to maintain correct posture and power.

Friction: stiffness of muscles, connective tissues and joints

The following will help reduce friction:
- Keep warm – Look at energy delivery systems.
- Hot bath or shower, sauna, hot climate and sunshine benefit many.
- Keep hydrated – Tennis players at Wimbledon always drink between games.
- Minerals for the right electrical properties – Hydrate with electrolyte
  solutions. My recipe is 2 g of salt plus 1 g of MMM (see page 72) in a litre

of water. This should be used by all athletes and during hot weather, fever or gastroenteritis. Also use in hot drinks – at this dilution one can hardly taste the salt.

- Transdermal minerals – This means of absorbing minerals is the basis of spa therapies, which have been popular for hundreds of years. Indeed, different spas have been traditionally used for a range of conditions, from arthritis to heart disease. Epsom salts from Epsom spa (magnesium sulphate) are excellent for arthritis. There may well be benefits from other spas and other minerals.
- Transdermal magnesium – I was initially sceptical about the benefits of transdermal magnesium because I could not see how such a tiny dose could have a therapeutic effect. However, the clinical benefits are profound – so many patients see benefit. Again remember Ovid: 'The result validates the deeds.'

Movement

MASSAGE AND MANIPULATION

My puppy dog, Nancy, stretches all her muscles after rest and before exercise. We humans should do the same. After exercise she loves to be stroked and massaged, sighing with pleasure. We humans should do the same. I think of this as ironing out the mechanical and electrical irregularities and restoring the normal frictions of connective tissue. There will be an outpouring of endogenous opiates from the brain. I cannot think of any medical condition that would not benefit from daily massage and the systemic anti-inflammatory, analgesic, feel-good factor that accompanies such.

SWIMMING AND HYDROTHERAPY

It is not difficult to see the benefit of giving joints, connective tissue and muscles the chance to heal and repair without gravity getting in the way. This, combined with the massaging effects of water, has wonderful healing properties. A hot seaside holiday offers so many health benefits: clean air; seafood; sunshine for vitamin D, mood and detox; water for swimming and transdermal minerals . . . the list goes on.

Wear and tear

Healing and repair of damaged tissues requires time (sleep and rest, page 227) and energy (see energy delivery mechanisms, page 21). It also requires raw materials. An old Chinese remedy for arthritis is to drink the broth of a twice-boiled chicken carcass. Of course, this contains all the raw materials of bone, connective tissue and muscle, which is a central part of cooking for the Paleo-ketogenic diet. Sanitised versions include glucosamine, methyl-sulphonyl-methane (MSM), chondroitin sulphate and hyaluronic acid, all of which are of proven benefit.

Minerals

In addition to the Basic Package, I regularly use these micronutrients:

- **Boron** – up to 20 mg daily.
- **Organic silica G5** – 30 ml daily. This was researched and developed by Dr Le Ribault. His discovery of the benefits of organic silica, followed by his persecution by the conventional medical establishment, is a must read: *The Persecution and Resistance of Loïc Le Ribault* by Martin Walker.
- **Strontium** – 250–500 mg daily is of proven benefit in osteoporosis. The NHS prescribable form of strontium is ranelate; this form does not occur naturally and so can be patented. I suspect side effects relate to the fact it is a ranelate. Furthermore the NHS prescription form is made up with the toxic sweetener aspartame. I use natural strontium chloride or carbonate 250–500 mg of elemental strontium daily. It requires an acid stomach for its absorption, so check for hypochlorhydria (see page 205).
- **Vitamin D** – up to 10,000 IU daily. This is highly protective against osteo-porosis for the above reasons. Vitamin D also improves muscular strength and balance, so one is less likely to fall over and break a bone.
- **Niacinamide** – 1,500–3,000 mg daily. In his book *The Common Cause of Joint Dysfunction published* in 1949, Dr William Kaufman carefully docu-mented the responses of 1,500 patients to niacinamide (a form of vitamin B3). What I found interesting was that all age groups, from children to octogenarians, responded – the older the patient, the better the response. Furthermore, it did not matter what the cause of the arthritis was – all responded equally well. I suspect this was because this vitamin improves energy delivery systems and so healing and repair were faster. There were no side effects.

I do not prescribe calcium. There is plenty of calcium in a Paleo-ketogenic diet. What is important is how well absorbed it is and whether it is dumped in the right place. Vitamin D improves calcium absorption from the gut and its deposition in bone. Furthermore, calcium and magnesium compete for absorption and the latter is arguably more important with respect to prevent-ing osteoporosis and certainly the commoner deficiency – taking high-dose calcium makes this imbalance even worse.

VII. Tools to treat abnormal growths
Reduce the total load of tumour cells
This can be done by surgery, radiotherapy or chemotherapy.

The Basic Package
Metabolic syndrome is a major risk factor for cancer. Cancers are evolution-arily primitive cells and can only survive on glucose. In this respect they are very much like yeast and rely entirely on anaerobic metabolism. Glucose is fermented in the absence of oxygen to produce energy. This is very ineffi-cient. Indeed, this inefficient burning of glucose probably explains the cancer cachexia (weight loss) seen in advanced cases.

Cells normally get the vast majority of their energy from mitochondria. This is extremely efficient; mitochondria can utilise not just glucose, but also energy from fat. These uses require oxygen. The reason it is important to understand this is because mitochondria control cell division. If mitochon-dria go slow and start to fail, this control is lost and the cell has the potential to turn into a cancerous cell. Heart cells, for example, have more mitochon-dria (25 per cent by weight) than any other cell in the body but cancer of the heart is rare. Cancers of muscle (20 per cent by weight mitochondria) are also rare.

The difference between a cancer cell and a normal cell, therefore, is how it gets its energy. By actively treating metabolic syndrome one starts to starve out the cancer cells. In this event, cancer cells up-grade the mechanism by which they absorb sugar, which is the same mechanism by which they absorb vitamin C – and vitamin C is toxic to cancer cells. This is the rationale that underpins taking vitamin C to bowel tolerance. This makes high-dose intravenous vita-min C a logical treatment.

Get rid of growth promoters
Growth promoters occur in Western cultures in at least four ways:

Dairy products – These are meant for fast-growing baby cows, so dairy prod-ucts contain growth promoters. These are naturally present in milk, but there may also be artificial growth promoters which are injected into cows to improve milk yields. I recommend *Your Life in Your Hands* by Professor Jane Plant who has shown that dairy products are associated with breast and prostate cancer. All dairy products are a problem for the same reasons, including goat and sheep. Organic dairy products may avoid the synthetic growth promoters but they do have natural growth promoters. Avoid these too.

Insulin is a growth promoter. Both type I and type II diabetics have an increased risk of cancer.

Obesity – Just carrying excessive adipose tissue results in higher levels of hormones, particularly oestrogen, and this too is a growth promoter.

Toxic chemicals – In particular, organochlorine and organophosphate pesticides, volatile organic compounds (VOCs) and toxic metals are carcinogenic. Test for these by fat biopsy, DNA adducts and toxic metal levels in urine following DMSA.

Improve antioxidant status

Free radicals are involved in carcinogenesis. These are highly reactive molecules with an unpaired electron so they 'stick' readily to almost anything and in doing so cause damage. Free radicals are inevitably produced as part of energy production and are used by the immune system to kill bacteria and viruses. However, too many are damaging and the body has a series of 'antioxidants' which mop up the free radicals to prevent excessive damage.

It is common to find extremely poor antioxidant status in cancer patients. This is partly because having poor antioxidant status is a major risk factor for developing cancer in the first place, and partly because the three main therapies used to treat cancer – namely surgery, chemotherapy and radiotherapy – produce an increased load of free radicals. Indeed, the mechanism by which radiotherapy and chemotherapy kill cancer cells is through the production of excessive free radicals. This is one of the ironies of these two treatments – they can create cancers as well as cure them. But all these excess free radicals further deplete antioxidants. Improving antioxidant status not only reduces one's chances of further tumours but also protects against the malign side effects of chemotherapy and radiotherapy.

At one stage there was concern that improving antioxidant status would block the beneficial effects of chemotherapy and radiotherapy, but there is little evidence that this is the case.

The three important frontline antioxidants, which in my view should be measured in every case, are: **superoxide dismutase, coenzyme Q10 and glutathione peroxidase**. These are present in microgram amounts. They will mop up excess electrons and pass them back to a second line of antioxidants, such as vitamin D, vitamin K, vitamin E, some of the B vitamins, lipoic acid, melatonin and many other such natural molecules, which then recycle the electron back to the ultimate repository of electrons, which is ascorbic acid. This makes vitamin C, of course, doubly important in the prevention and treatment of cancer. There are many natural antioxidants in foods, hence the importance of eating vegetables, nuts, seeds and berries. (Do not eat large amounts of sweet fruit since fructose is a sugar with the potential to ferment.)

Vitamin D merits a special mention. Vitamin D is highly protective against cancer. The best source is sunshine – not so much that you burn (which causes free-radical damage to the skin) but enough to make you tan. There is a clear relationship between sunshine exposure and risk of cancer – that is, the more sunshine you can get without actually burning, the more you are protected from getting cancer.

Address causes of, and reduce, inflammation

Many cancers are triggered and driven by chronic inflammation, which may be driven by infection, autoimmunity, toxic stress or radiation. Causes to be aware of include:

Viruses – cervical cancer (HPV), hepatoma (hepatitis B), Kaposi's
   sarcoma (HIV), Hodgkins' disease (Epstein-Barr virus) and Burkitt's
   lymphoma (Epstein-Barr virus) and others
Bacteria – *Helicobacter pylori* (stomach cancer), chronic dental infection
   (oral cancer) and others
Upper fermenting gut, Crohn's disease and ulcerative colitis are
   microbe driven and risk factors for cancer
Tuberculosis increases the risk of lung cancer
Mastitis increases the risk of breast cancer
Autoimmune systemic sclerosis increases the risk of lung cancer five-fold
Coeliac disease increases the risk of lymphoma
Hashimoto's thyroiditis increases the risk of thyroid cancer

Often the trigger is multifactorial, with multiple risk factors having a cock-tail effect. Smoking is good at triggering all sorts of cancers because smoke is an irritant, contains toxic carcinogens and increases the risk of an infection. Many lung cancers are triggered by polluting industry which discharges into the atmosphere a range of toxic metals, noxious gases, VOCs, pesticides and radiation. These are emitted as such small particles that they are invisible.

Interestingly, allergy is mildly protective against cancer. Perhaps allergy systems developed as part of our defence against cancer?

Improve energy delivery systems

Improve mitochondrial, thyroid and adrenal function.

Monitor the effects of treatment

Many tumours have a tumour marker detectable in the blood. The one best known is prostate-specific antigen (PSA) for prostate cancer. But many tumours have similar markers which are very useful for monitoring how effective treatment has been. Sequential testing can show if one is winning or losing the battle against cancer and give some guidance as to how hard one has to work at the regimes.

VIII. Tools of the trade: sex hormones

Sex hormones are essential for procreation, and that is essential for the survival of our genes. But having high levels of sex hormones is a risky business. Being a fertile female and becoming pregnant is potentially dangerous.

I never prescribe female sex hormones because I believe there is overwhelming evidence that they are damaging to health in the long term. In the short term they suppress symptoms without addressing the root cause of problems. It does not matter if such hormones are natural or synthetic, given as pills, patches or injections, their toxic actions are extensions of their physiological actions. These physiological actions are to:

Raise blood sugar levels – This is essential to protect the baby from hypoglycaemia but may result in the 'diabetes of pregnancy'.

Raise blood pressure and thicken blood vessels – Again, this is to nourish the baby. However, it puts the mother at risk of arterial disease and stroke.

Immuno-suppress – This is essential to prevent the baby being rejected immunologically because effectively the baby is a foreign body. However, this puts the mother at increased risk of infection. This is a particular problem for women on the Pill and who have, or may be at risk of, sexually transmitted diseases. In this connection, I believe the Pill and HRT are major risk factors for CFS.

Immuno-dysregulate – Women taking female sex hormones are at greater risk of autoimmunity and allergy.

Promote growth – Again, this action is essential to allow the breasts, ovaries and womb to grow in preparation for pregnancy, but growth promotion is one step away from cancer. Female sex hormones have been classified as class one carcinogens by the World Health Organisation. Established cancer is an absolute contra-indication for female sex hormones.

Make blood more sticky – Again, this action is essential to staunch haemorrhage during birth, but it puts mothers at greater risk of deep vein thrombosis (DVT) and pulmonary embolus.

Testosterone – I am ambivalent about prescribing testosterone. I believe that low levels in younger men are the result of poor micronutrients, poor diet, inadequate physical exercise, toxic stress and other such. I don't think testosterone is harmful if used in physiological doses and may well be an acquired metabolic dyslexia (see page 190). We know testosterone levels fall with age so logically many men could benefit from low-dose, doctor-monitored supplementation.

IX. Potentially dangerous tools – Doctors, prescription drugs, vaccinations, and medical investigations

Physician, heal thyself [and leave the rest of us alone!]

LUKE 4.23, The Bible, King James Version (adapted!)

After cancer and heart disease, the most common cause of death in modern Western society is the medical profession – drug side effects, medical investigations, and doctors' mistakes (including sloppy hand-writing). Indeed, when doctors go on strike (Israel, New York, Columbia, Los Angeles and others) the death rate falls by up to 50 per cent. Hospitals are dangerous places with the potential to pass on infections (MRSA, *Clostridium difficile* and others). Malnutrition, dehydration, chronic insomnia, lack of physical exercise and sunshine together with social isolation erode resistance to disease and ability to heal.

After 20 years of NHS practice I left partly because I felt I did not have the clinical freedoms I required to practise to the standards I wanted within the constraints of the NHS. Indeed, at one stage I was reprimanded because my prescribing costs were too low and therefore I was considered to be a bad doctor!

My greatest concerns are as follows:

Symptom-suppressing medication – We have symptoms for good reason – to protect us from ourselves. Taking such medication gives patients the false impression that they are tackling the root causes of problems and so mislead them and give a false sense of security. Pain killers allow us to use limbs which should be rested. People taking non-steroidal anti-inflammatories or paracetamol for arthritis require joint replacement surgery sooner. Anti-inflammatories allow us to work through colds and influenzas when rest is called for – so increasing the risk of post-viral chronic fatigue syndrome. Drugs to suppress fever, vomiting, diarrhoea, coughing, rhinitis, etc prevent us reducing our load of infectious organism. We know infectious microbes drive many disease processes, such as allergy, CFS/ME, autoimmunity and cancer.

Use of the Pill and HRT – These have increased rates of cancer, infertility, metabolic syndrome and its complications, allergy, autoimmunity and CFS/ME.

Vaccinations – These may have the potential to do good, but they also have the potential to harm. There is good evidence to show that vaccinations may be a major cause of modern epidemics of autoimmunity (such as type I diabetes in children), allergy (including asthma), autism, CFS/ME and possibly dementia. I recommend the book *The Truth about Vaccinations* by NHS GP Dr Richard Halvorsen, which is essential reading for any parent.

Acid blockers such as proton pump inhibitors, H2 blockers and antacids – An acid stomach is vital to protect against infection, to absorb minerals and to digest protein. Acid blockers put us at risk of gastroenteritis, food poisoning and gut viruses, including glandular fever, osteoporosis and allergy (because undigested protein molecules present an antigenically interesting load). They also put us at risk of upper fermenting gut which, I suspect, is in its turn a major risk factor for cancers of the stomach, oesophagus and possibly colon.

Asthma inhalers – Prior to these drugs becoming available, wheezy bronchitis (the old name for asthma) was an uncommon and mild self-limiting condition. Children grew out of it. Now that the blue and the brown inhalers are routinely prescribed, asthma has become chronic. It appears that beta-agonists, and perhaps steroid inhalers, upset the normal immune mechanisms for switching off allergies. They seem to make the wheezy bronchitis permanent. They certainly detract from the important business of identifying the underlying causes of asthma and treating from first principles.

Overuse of antibiotics and antifungals – As a result of many of the above issues and failings, antibiotics and antifungals are often prescribed. There is no doubt they have their place and I would hate to practise medicine without them, but the more we use them the more likely it becomes that resistant strains of microbe will appear until we face the nightmare scenario of widespread antibiotic resistance. Already this is a problem in hospitals with MRSA. This problem can only get worse.

Statins – Drug companies are running out of patentable money makers and now have to generate diseases in order to create sales. A successful propaganda programme now has Westerners believing that a high-fat diet results in high cholesterol which results in arterial and heart disease. What a joke!

Even doctors have been so brain-washed and dish out statins like Smarties at a child's party. Not only is the propaganda untrue, but statins do not exert any benefits through reducing cholesterol levels. We know biochemically that any benefits arise because they are vitamin D mimics. But statins inhibit endogenous production of coenzyme Q10 and so could be expected to accelerate the ageing process with its attendant risks of heart failure, dementia and cancer.

Beta blockers – These block the effect of adrenalin. In the short term, they control some symptoms of stress, but in the long term they accelerate many of the features of metabolic syndrome, such as diabetes.

Roaccutane – This is a drug used for treating acne. It is metabolised in the body into a drug which is also used for cancer chemotherapy. I have seen patients with serious mood disturbances after taking this drug, including two young men who subsequently committed suicide.

Many prescription drugs are addictive – Doctors do not seem to have woken up to the addictive nature of modern Western diets and lifestyles and fail to recognise that in prescribing many drugs they are simply replacing one addiction with another, or adding to the addictive load. It is clear to the untrained observer that the occupants of psychiatric wards are blatant addicts, controlling their stress with sugar, refined carbohydrates, tea, coffee, nicotine and, on escape, alcohol, cannabis and other such. SSRIs (serotonin re-uptake inhibitors – the most-used antidepressants) were promoted on the back of not being addictive, but this is untrue – many of my patients develop severe withdrawal symptoms when they try to stop them. Major tranquillisers, like chlorpromazine and haloperidol, result in metabolic syndrome and all associated risks.

Medical investigations involving radiation – Radiation is an obvious cause of cancer and the medical profession is responsible for large doses. There is now increasing concern that the possible benefits of mammography are outweighed by the damaging effects of radiation. I believe that mammography will soon be abandoned as a screening tool for breast cancer for reasons given in the book *Mammography Screening: Truth, Lies and Controversy* by Dr Peter Gotzsche. See www.cochrane.dk.

Doses of drugs – Any drugs which inhibit enzyme systems, and this is most of them, may be toxic. Getting the dose right is critical and, indeed, many deaths occur because of sloppy hand-writing so that the wrong dose is dispensed. Drug interactions increase exponentially as more drugs are prescribed. The *British National Formulary*, the 'drug bible', lists reactions between any two drugs, but there is no such list for three or more.[12] By contrast, *nutritional supplements* work by facilitating enzyme systems and so they work more efficiently. This means the potential for error is miniscule.

Conclusion

I hope by now you will have the confidence and determination to identify your symptoms and apply the tools of the trade to correct those symptoms using benign but proven interventions. However, many people start with clinical pictures and diseases and this is the subject of the next chapter.

CHAPTER 4

Treatment – the choice of tools for particular diseases

In this chapter, I identify specific diseases, along with their underlying causes, and target them with particular tools. I have grouped the diseases into 'like' conditions according to their causes and structured the chapter under the following six headings:

I. The general approach to avoiding and treating all disease:
Ageing – how to stay well and live to one's full potential
Fatigue – CFS/ME versus peak performance

II. Conditions collectively known as 'metabolic syndrome': an inevitable result of Western diets and lifestyles, resulting in degeneration, which is characterised by:
Hypertension (high blood pressure)
Obesity
Diabetes
Arteriosclerosis
Mental problems: anxiety, obsessive compulsive disorders, eating disorders, depression
Cholesterol
Constipation
Diverticulosis
Osteoporosis
Eye disease: macular degeneration, glaucoma, cataracts

III. **Conditions driven by the long-term effects of metabolic syndrome and inflammation:**
Heart disease
Heart attack
Stroke
Cancer
Dementia and prion disorders: Alzheimer's, Parkinson's, motor neurone disease, CJD
Gynaecological problems: polycystic ovarian syndrome (PCOS), irregular periods, menorrhagia, infertility

IV. **Conditions associated with inflammation:**
Autoimmunity
Anaphylaxis
Asthma, chronic obstructive airway's disease (COAD/COPD), rhinitis, sinusitis, ENT problems
Eczema and urticaria
Psoriasis
Acne and rosacea
Irritable bowel syndrome, GERD, ulcers
Migraine and headache
Inflammatory bowel disease: Crohn's disease, ulcerative colitis
Irritable bladder syndrome, interstitial cystitis
Joint, connective tissue and muscle problems

V. **Preconception care and afterwards:**
Pregnancy
Paediatrics

VI. **Twenty-first century syndromes resulting from increasing environmental pollution:**
Mercury poisoning
Sick building syndrome
Gulf War syndrome
Sheep dip 'flu
Aerotoxic syndrome
9/11 syndrome
Silicone implant syndrome
Wind turbine syndrome

I. The general approach to avoiding and treating all disease

Prevention is better than Cure.

OLD ENGLISH PROVERB of unknown origin

Modern Western lifestyles are driven by addiction and this is very damaging to health. People go through life on an addictive ladder which starts in childhood with carbohydrates, refined sugars and dairy products. These are consumed in an addictive way. There is then an escalation of addiction as young people move onto chocolate, caffeine, alcohol, nicotine, and then up to cannabis, ecstasy, cocaine and heroin. It is very obvious that these latter substances are addictive and damaging to health and so long as the Grim Reaper does not intervene, people recognise this and move back down the addictive ladder. However, everybody gets stuck on the first rung, which is addiction to sugars and refined carbohydrate. These substances (because I do not like to call them 'foods') are not generally perceived to be addictive – indeed, they are not just socially acceptable, but desirable – we express our love for others with such junk food.

I can resist anything but temptation.

OSCAR WILDE (1854–1900)

Junk food is addictive because it spikes blood sugar levels and the rate at which the blood sugar increases results in a hit in the brain of neurotransmitters that have a calming effect. Indeed, we call this 'comfort eating'. This emotional–psychological attachment to junk food clouds logical, rational thought which tells us that we should not be eating it. It is sugars and refined carbohydrates that are driving our present epidemics of cancer, heart disease, diabetes and dementia. I do not need to look into a crystal ball to tell such Westerners what they are going to die from but I can also tell them what they will suffer on the way – namely, fatigue, obesity, diabetes, mental disorders, rotten teeth, arthritis and osteoporosis!

Addiction is not just about food – it extends to gambling, sex, money, fuel and power. I am fascinated by the history of the English-speaking people, but it is clear to me that much of this was driven by addiction. I could never understand why the West Indies were so important to Britain until I appreciated the massive proportion of our business that came from trade involving these islands; that trade involved the major addictions – namely, sugar, tobacco, caffeine, alcohol and, dare I say it, energy in the form of the slave trade.

Addictions cause many other problems downstream – not just the obvious psychological problems, but, for example, the fermenting gut; much more of this later.

Evolution gives us the principles to achieve good health. Good health was essential for survival of the fittest. We evolved in tribes, caring for family members, running naked under the Equatorial sun, initially gathering abundant shellfish and fish on the coasts, then migrating and surviving the Ice Age as carnivores when we fostered dogs for sentry duty and hunting. Being physically active meant eating large amounts of organic food with high levels of micronutrients.

Modern Western society life often involves junk food, which is calorie-rich and micronutrient-poor, being physically idle because we can, shielded from sunshine and light, exposed to a range of toxic chemicals, and often living in social isolation, chronically sleep deprived. We are seeing a temporary and unsustainable survival of the unfit and fattest.

I want the best of both worlds – the stimulus, interest and luxuries of modern life together with those interventions that respect evolutionary principles. The starting point for staying well, preventing and treating any disease condition is the 'Basic Package'. This Basic Package is what we should all be putting in place all the time. It is a blueprint for good health. I spend more time talking about this Basic Package than all other subjects put together. Once the Basic Package is in place, everything else follows relatively easily and logically. It is really no good leaping to esoteric treatments with high-dose nutritional supplements, herbals, prescription medication, detox regimes, or whatever, without first putting this in place.

The Basic Package

The Basic Package is what we should all be doing all the time – see Chapter 3 (page 65):

   I. Paleo-ketogenic diet
  II. Multivitamins, minerals, essential fatty acids
 III. Sleep
  IV. Exercise
   V. Sunshine and daylight
  VI. Reduction of the chemical burden
 VII. Sufficient physical and mental security to satisfy our universal need to love and care, and be loved and cared for
VIII. Avoidance of infections and treat aggressively

Ageing – how to stay well and live to one's full potential

Youth is wasted on the young.

OSCAR WILDE (1854–1900)

When I was a boy of 14, my father was so ignorant I could hardly stand to have the old man around. But when I got to be 21, I was astonished at how much the old man had learned in seven years.

MARK TWAIN (1835–1910)

With age, you can stay just as fit and just as well but you have to work harder at it. Once we have had our children, we are on the evolutionary scrap-heap. No matter if we die – the Olympic flame of DNA has been passed on to the next generation! This means that to stay fit and well we have to be clever.

As we age, the imperative to do the Basic Package becomes more powerful. Indeed, as we age and our biochemistry slows down, we may need more substrate to achieve the same result – that is, more micronutrients. I suspect 'acquired metabolic dyslexias' (see page 190) become a feature – we become less good at making certain key molecules and we should supplement these.

Acquired problems

It is **mitochondria** that determine the ageing process and so a package of supplements to feed mitochondria, together with detox regimes to reduce mitochondrial inhibition, will allow mitochondria to function to their full potential – theoretically, about 120 years.

Gut function declines and so we become less efficient at digesting and absorbing food. We often develop an **upper fermenting gut** and all the problems that accompany such. I suspect upper fermenting gut is the major cause of oesophageal and stomach cancer.

In our modern polluted world we bio-accumulate **toxins** in flesh and fat and they may get to a critical level that triggers a problem. **Type II diabetes** we know is partly due to this problem – there is plenty of insulin, but the insulin receptor is blocked by pollutants. We call it insulin resistance. These toxins include heavy metals, pesticides and volatile organic compounds (VOCs) – so-called persistent organic pollutants (POPs). Many POPs are known to trigger cancer and prion disorders (such as Alzheimer's disease, Parkinson's disease and motor neurone disease). I think of prion disorders as **protein cancers**.

Our ability to synthesise **hormones** declines and physiological supplements of adrenal hormones, melatonin and possibly thyroid hormones and testosterone may be helpful. I do not agree with supplementing oestrogen and progesterone as HRT because, being growth promoters, they are carcinogenic. I believe the Pill and HRT are major causes of current epidemics of breast cancer.

We become more prone to disease associated with **inflammation** – often useless inflammation as in autoimmunity and allergy – and inflammation is damaging. Do not start with anti-inflammatory drugs; identify the cause! **Metabolic syndrome** is a major driver of inflammation.

How we can tackle them

As we age, in order of priority, we should:

- Work even harder at the Basic Package. In particular, reduce carbohydrate intake to prevent problems of the upper fermenting gut.
- Learn to pace activity so that energy demands can easily be met by energy delivery.
- Use tools to improve energy delivery – the most important supplements to support mitochondria are: coenzyme Q10 (250 mg daily), vitamin B3 as niacinamide (500 mg daily), D-ribose (5 g daily) and acetyl L-carnitine (500 mg daily).
- Take trans-dermal vitamin B12 (1 mg daily, or ideally a B12 injection 2 mg monthly).
- Do tests for thyroid and adrenal function every five years.
- Detoxify using the best tools for detoxification – supplements to facilitate detoxification such as glutathione (250 mg daily); regular heating and showering regimes to reduce toxic load (either intense exercise or sauna-ing); consider tests to look for toxic load, such as DNA adducts, toxic metals in urine following a chelating agent and possibly fat biopsy to measure body burdens of pesticides and VOCs.
- Deal with a fermenting gut – tools to tackle the fermenting gut include, possibly, use of digestive aids such as betaine hydrochloride and pancreatic enzymes. Take vitamin C (5 grams or more, to bowel tolerance), last thing at night to reduce microbial numbers.
- Be increasingly wary of symptom-suppressing medication which has the potential to accelerate underlying disease processes.

Fatigue

> *I am somewhat exhausted; I wonder how a battery feels when it pours electricity into a non-conductor?*
>
> Sir Arthur Conan Doyle (1859–1930)

Fatigue is an essential symptom which we all experience – it protects the body from itself. Without fatigue we would quickly use up all our reserves of energy, have no rest time to allow for healing and repair, and rapidly succumb. Fatigue is relative – we could all put in place interventions to improve energy levels, but they are hard work – the principles that underlie treatment for CFS apply equally to those with better levels of energy and, indeed, elite athletes.

Stress is the symptom we experience when the brain knows it does not have the energy/resources to deal with demand – which may be mental, physical, emotional, financial, infectious or whatever. Part of being robust and well is ensuring that there are always sufficient energy reserves to deal with the unexpected, so do not live life on the edge! Do not live life like Vincent in the film *Gattaca* where he says that:

> *You want to know how I did it? This is how I did it, Anton: I never saved anything for the swim back.*

> VINCENT, *Gattaca* (1997)

The mechanisms by which causes of metabolic syndrome are associated with fatigue result from a multiplicity of effects on energy delivery mechanisms and pro-inflammatory effects.

Treatment of fatigue

- The Basic Package.
- Extras as per treatment of ageing, including tools to tackle energy delivery systems: mitochondrial, thyroid, adrenal and gut function.
- Identify how energy is wasted: identify and treat the immunological and emotional holes in the energy bucket.

Further details of treating CFS/ME, together with the science that underpins such, can be seen in my first book *Diagnosis and Treatment of Chronic Fatigue Syndrome: it's mitochondria, not hypochondria.*

II. Conditions collectively known as 'metabolic syndrome'

Metabolic syndrome is a clinical picture comprised of one or all of the following: loss of control of blood sugar, obesity and hypertension, all resulting in arteriosclerosis.

Symptoms of metabolic syndrome

Early symptoms of metabolic syndrome include:
- Fatigue – in particular, inability to get fit
- Foggy brain – such as poor scholastic performance in children, possibly even dyslexia
- High BMI
- Upper fermenting gut resulting in irritable bowel syndrome
- Central obesity – because the immune system is busy in the gut either for reasons of allergy or the upper fermenting gut
- Inability to deal with stress
- Insomnia

Medium-term symptoms include:
- Mental disease, such as eating disorders (anorexia, bulimia), PMT, obsessive compulsive disorder, anxiety and depression
- Gum disease, dental decay and tooth loss
- A pro-thrombotic tendency (such as deep vein thrombosis – DVT)
- Osteoarthritis, muscle aches and pains
- Polycystic ovarian syndrome, irregular periods, menorrhagia and infertility
- Kidney malfunction with falling eGFR (estimated glomerular filtration rate) or protein in urine
- Premature ageing

Late symptoms include:
- Type II diabetes
- Arteriosclerosis, strokes and heart disease
- Eye disease – cataracts, macular degeneration and glaucoma
- Major mental disease, perhaps including psychosis
- Peripheral neuropathy
- Dementia due to arteriosclerosis ('type III diabetes')
- Dementia due to prion diseases, such as Alzheimer's disease
- Prion disorders, such as Parkinson's disease, and possibly motor neurone disease
- Kidney failure
- Possibly deafness

Tests may show:
- Raised levels of triglycerides
- High levels of LDL cholesterol (unfriendly) and low HDL cholesterol (friendly)

- High fasting glucose; abnormal glucose tolerance tests
- Non-alcoholic fatty liver disease
- High-normal ESR (erythrocyte sedimentation rate is a test for inflammation; the 'normal' range has been moved upwards recently since so many 'normal' people have metabolic syndrome) – the ESR should be below 10
- Low-normal estimated glomerular filtration rate (eGFR – from poor kidney function)

However, the early stages of metabolic syndrome may not show any abnormal tests. It is a clinical diagnosis.

Causes

Metabolic syndrome results from five interlinking strands:
- Modern Western diets which are high in sugar and refined carbohydrates, with allergenic and growth-promoting foods
- Modern Western diets which are deficient in micronutrients – minerals, vitamins and essential fatty acids
- Toxic stress from the outside world (toxic metals, volatile organic compounds and pesticides, collectively known as persistent organic pollutants, or POPs)
- Toxic stress from the upper fermenting gut and unwelcome food additives
- Lack of physical and mental exercise

Dogs and cats also suffer from metabolic syndrome. The evolutionarily correct food for our beloved dogs and cats is raw meat, fish and eggs. By feeding them cooked tinned meat full of cereals, with biscuits, we are inducing metabolic syndrome. Cats and dogs now become overweight, diabetic, and develop heart disease, cancer and degenerative conditions. They have adopted human diets and diseases.

Treatment of metabolic syndrome

The Basic Package – see page 67.

Hypertension (high blood pressure)

Chronologically there are two phases. High blood pressure results when the arteries narrow. This occurs when the stress hormone adrenaline is released. In other words, stress causes high blood pressure. That we know, but what we overlook is the commonest cause of stress, which is wobbly blood sugar levels. The rate at which blood sugar rises determines the amount of insulin released; this triggers a precipitate fall in blood sugar. The brain then goes into panic mode because it is about to run out of fuel and stimulates release of adrenaline in order to kick the liver to release glucose stores and restore blood sugar levels. The rate at which blood sugar falls determines the amount of adrenaline released. However, this also increases blood pressure.

Adrenaline causes the symptoms of low blood sugar and makes us feel stressed; it is, of course, the stress hormone. We resolve this by comfort-eating sugar and refined carbohydrates thereby perpetuating the vicious cycle.

The problem with arteries narrowing and blood pressure rising is that the flow of blood becomes more turbulent, especially where arteries divide. This damages the delicate lining of the arterial wall. This damage is amplified by sugar, toxins in cigarette smoke, heavy metals, pesticides and other such – this may be the mechanism by which homocysteine causes arteriosclerosis.

This brings us to the second phase. Damage has to be repaired by the immune system and this involves inflammation. The immune system creates a patch, which in the longer term is replaced by scar tissue, which contracts and stiffens the arterial wall. This patch is called arteriosclerosis. The artery becomes stiff and narrowed as scar tissue is laid down.

The first phase of adrenaline-induced hypertension is reversible as adrenaline levels fall. Blood pressure is variable. At this stage much can be done to normalise blood pressure by addressing the causes of adrenaline release – largely diet.

After years of the first phase, the second phase cuts in. Arteries become stiff and permanently narrowed. Typically there is a wide pulse pressure which can be seen in blood pressure readings. By this stage it is more difficult to normalise blood pressure through diet and lifestyle changes, although it is never too late to start!

Treatment of high blood pressure

- Routine blood and urine tests to exclude pathology, such as kidney and thyroid disease.
- The Basic Package.
- Reduce adrenaline release – eat a Paleo-ketogenic diet with a low glycaemic index (GI); this stops the adrenaline release that accompanies hypoglycaemia. Address other causes of adrenaline release, such as lifestyle stressors: lack of sleep, psychological, emotional, financial and so on.

- Exercise – This is known to reduce blood pressure by several possible mechanisms, including the metabolic glycogen sponge, helping to detox, the feel-good factor, improved sleep and so on.
- Reduce vasospasm (any condition in which a blood vessel's spasm leads to vasoconstriction) resulting from other mechanisms.
- Address magnesium deficiency (see page 81).
- Address allergies to foods and chemicals (such as pesticides) – these can present with vasospasm and high blood pressure.
- Reduce endogenous toxic damage to arteries that results in arteriosclerosis:

    Sugar is directly toxic to arteries by sticking to membranes and causing AGEs (advanced glycation end products). This is further reason to follow a low GI diet.

    Homocysteine – High levels result from a slow methylation cycle. Take the standard package of nutritional supplements and the package of supplements to correct the methylation cycle.

- Address exogenous toxic problems – Check heavy metals in urine after taking a chelating agent (DMSA). Consider fat biopsy to look for toxic load.
- Treat any condition associated with inflammation.

Inflammation may result from infection, allergy or autoimmunity. If it is present generally in the blood, this damages arteries because of free radical activity. Inflammation in the blood is measured by markers such as ESR, C-reactive protein and plasma viscosity. Any inflammatory condition, such as rheumatoid arthritis or inflammatory bowel disease, must be treated, if only to reduce this dangerous and useless inflammation.

Obesity

> She looked as if she had been poured into her clothes and forgotten to say when.
>
> PG WODEHOUSE (1881–1975)

The simple paradigm, adopted by most doctors, that obesity is a simple case of overeating and under exercising has clearly failed Westerners. In order of importance obesity is caused by:

Addiction to junk food – We use addiction to cope with stress, and the commonest, cheapest and most socially acceptable addiction is sugar and refined carbohydrates. We call this junk food. In other words, we deal with stress by comfort-eating. One effective way to lose weight is to swap to another addiction, such as smoking – but health-wise you are no better off! Eating junk food, in an addictive way, results in high levels of blood sugar and high levels of insulin. Insulin brings blood sugar down by shunting it into fat; this mechanism is so effective that people can eat very low-calorie diets, but still not lose weight. This is because those diets are carbohydrate based, so high insulin results and the hormonal drive is constantly to resist fats being mobilised for energy production.

Low-calorie diets result in poor fuel delivery to mitochondria, so people feel tired, lethargic, cold and depressed. Life becomes a misery, with thoughts of food constantly at the front of the mind. Low-calorie diets are not sustainable in the long term and lead to yo-yo weight changes.

Stress – This draws people to addiction to cope with that stress. Work and emotional and psychological stress are usually obvious. A common overlooked stress is lack of sleep.

Food craving because of allergy to food – One of the odd results of allergy is that people get addicted to their allergen and allergic to their addiction! Allergy and addiction seem to be two sides of the same coin. If you eat an excessive amount of a food (for example, gluten grains – bread, pasta, pastry, biscuit) or dairy products (milk, cheese, yoghurt, butter, cream) then cutting that food out may help. Where there are food allergies there is often allergic oedema and people commonly lose up to half a stone of weight over a few days when they stop consuming problem foods. Eat a Paleo-ketogenic diet.

The fermenting gut exacerbates a hypoglycaemic tendency (see page 201). I have much to learn with regard to probiotics, but we know that gut flora has a direct impact on weight. The mechanism for this I have yet to discover.

Food craving because of micronutrient deficiency – This is most obvious in pregnancy where there are increased demands for micronutrients. Take the standard package of nutritional supplements.

Poor energy delivery – Due to poor mitochondrial, thyroid and adrenal function one may be unable to burn fuel. Many of my CFS/ME patients struggle to lose weight. Borderline hypothyroidism is very common and unrecognised by the medical profession. The thyroid is the accelerator pedal of our metabolic engines (mitochondria) so all metabolism goes slow with low-calorie use.

Toxic stress – In the short term, the body can deal with fat-soluble toxins by dumping them in fat. The problem with weight loss is that these toxins are mobilised into the blood stream, potentially resulting in acute poisoning.

When I measure pesticide levels in fat the result is in milligrams per kilogram whereas blood results are in micrograms – that is, a thousand-fold difference. So far I have never failed to find pesticides in any fat sample. Sauna/heating detox regimes help to bring toxins out through the skin and reduce the systemic poisoning. The body protects itself from poisoning through a metabolic reluctance to mobilise fats – I do not yet know the mechanism by which this is achieved.

Lack of exercise – The reason men burn more calories than women is because they have a larger muscle mass and this requires more calories at rest to maintain it. This also means they are warmer than women. The business of exercising does not burn many calories. However, muscle mass at rest needs more energy to maintain it. Muscle mass is increased by the right sort of exercise which gets one into anaerobic metabolism with lactic acid burn (see page 46).

Inflammation – The body dumps fat (for fuel) where the immune system is active. This explains why people who are apple-shaped are at greater risk of heart disease, because the immune system is active in the gut – for reasons of either allergy or the upper fermenting gut. The male beer belly is caused by fermenting gut. Metabolic syndrome is partly diagnosed from waist size.

Sex hormones – The Pill and HRT induce metabolic syndrome by allowing a high blood sugar and encouraging deposition of fat. Sex hormones are an essential part of pregnancy to ensure adequate nourishment of the growing baby. However, this is at the expense of the mother, who suffers increased risk of metabolic syndrome, diabetes, hypertension (eclampsia), cancer and psychological problems.

Treatment of obesity

- The Basic Package (see page 67) – In particular, low GI diet, low-allergen diet and environment, sleep and the right sort of exercise.
- Tools to treat energy delivery – Think mitochondria, thyroid and adrenal function.
- Detoxification regimes.
- Avoid the Pill and HRT.
- For two days a week eat a very low-calorie diet. This mimics evolutionary principles – primitive man did not eat three regular meals a day. The idea is that calorie burning is closely tied to calorie intake. However, there is a time lag of at least one day before calorie burning falls commensurate with intake. So if, for example, normal intake is 2,000 calories a day, and there is one day of 500 calories, then 1,500 calories worth of fat will be lost. After the one day, return to normal 2,000 calorie intake but then repeat, say, twice a week.

Diabetes*

Type I diabetes is an autoimmune disease – see treatment of autoimmunity, page 150. However, putting in place the package of treatment for type II diabetes is additionally helpful and should reduce insulin requirements. Indeed, going into the new regime must be done slowly and blood sugars monitored carefully for obvious reasons.

Type II diabetes is an inevitable result of modern Western diets and lifestyles. Indeed, at the present rate of increase, by the year 2030 50 per cent of the Western population will be diabetic. The four aspects that need most attention are diet, micronutrient deficiency, exercise and toxic stress.

What is so interesting is that in type II diabetes one might expect to see low insulin levels. Actually, the reverse is the case – these are normal or high. Even the conventional doctors recognise this, and having type II diabetes is described as being insulin resistant. Insulin is present, but the insulin receptor is blocked. This issue was flagged up by a paper in *The Lancet*, which looked at the levels of persistent organic pollutants (POPs) in the general population.[13] What they found was that those with the highest levels of POPs, compared with those with the lowest level, were 38 times more likely to be diabetic.

Treatment of diabetes

- As per the treatment of obesity (see page 133) – Obesity and type II diabetes often coexist for the same reasons. **Exercise** is particularly important to encourage the muscle and liver metabolic sponge to more efficiently mop up blood sugar spikes.
- Additional micronutrients that are particularly important in blood sugar control, most notably vitamin B3 and chromium. I would suggest niacinamide (slow release, 1,500 mg), chromium (300 mcg), zinc (20 mg) daily in addition to the Basic Package.
- Tools to tackle toxic load – Do a fat biopsy for pesticides and volatile organic compounds (VOCs) and measure toxic metals in urine after taking the chelating agent DMSA. Do appropriate detox regimes (see page 105).

---

* **Historical note:** The word 'diabetes' derives from the Ancient Greek word for 'siphon'. An Ancient Greek physician noted that patients with diabetes urinated excessively, 'siphoning' fluid out of their bodies. The full name of the condition we commonly call 'diabetes' is 'diabetes mellitus', mellitus being Latin for 'honey-sweet', since the patient's urine was noticeably sweet. There is an unrelated condition, 'diabetes insipidus', that causes excessive urination as well, but here urine is dilute (very pale) and has no taste. The Latin word 'insipidus' means tasteless.

Established type II diabetics must be careful whilst adopting the above regimes: they are highly effective, blood sugar levels will fall and there may be no further need for medication. Blood sugar must be carefully monitored.

Type I diabetics may well be able to reduce their dose of insulin but can never stop insulin injections completely.

Arteriosclerosis

Aterteriosclerosis is an inevitable result of modern Western diets and lifestyles. Indeed, the earliest lesions of arteriosclerosis we now see in young children.

Arteries are damaged by high blood pressure, high blood sugar and exogenous toxins – especially heavy metals (smoking), pesticides and VOCs – but also by cancer chemotherapy, endogenous toxins (such as homocysteine and possibly products of the fermenting gut) and inflammation.

Arteries are damaged by inflammation so it is important to identify the causes, which may be allergic or autoimmune.

Magnesium is particularly important in arterial disease and treatment of such, using Dr Sam Browne's regime of intravenous magnesium – 2–6 ml of intravenous magnesium sulphate, 50 per cent given as a bolus injection over 1–2 minutes every day to once monthly – is highly effective.

Treatment of arteriosclerosis

- Treat as for metabolic syndrome (see page 121).
- Treat blood pressure as above (see page 130).
- Treat blood sugar as for diabetes (see page 134).
- Identify and use tools to treat pro-inflammatory problems, especially the upper fermenting gut. Test for, and correct, antioxidant status (see page 43).
- Identify and, where appropriate, address toxic load (see page 105). Toxic metals are a common cause of arterial damage, as is homocysteine.
- Have intravenous magnesium injections.

Mental problems: anxiety, obsessive compulsive disorders, eating disorders, depression

We are seeing epidemics of mental problems, which are an inevitable result of modern Western diets and lifestyles. I suspect these are another unforeseen manifestation of metabolic syndrome – the effects of such on the brain. Indeed, these symptoms may well be the forerunners of more serious mental disorders, including psychosis and dementia. Alzheimer's disease, for example, has been dubbed 'type III diabetes of the brain' (although this is a misnomer – the actual pathology of that type of dementia is atherosclerotic; true Alzheimer's is a prion disorder [see page 62]). The use of this terminology reflects the power of Western high-carbohydrate diets to cause dementia.

In mental disorders, addiction prevails. This is admirably demonstrated by the manner in which Sir Winston Churchill dealt with his depression, which he referred to as his 'Black Dog'. Churchill drank vast quantities of alcohol, as approved by his doctor, ate large quantities of his favourite stilton cheese and also indulged in rich desserts. In addition, of course, he smoked his beloved imported cigars, for which he had developed a taste as a teenager.

Sufferers are mentally stressed and turn to addiction to control that stress. This often starts with sugar and refined carbohydrates, moves on to nicotine and alcohol, and then to serious drugs of abuse – cannabis, cocaine, heroin, etc. An essential part of treatment is to squeeze out all the addictions.

Modern psychiatrists do not seem to recognise this addiction problem. Indeed, their treatments with minor tranquillisers, major tranquillisers and antidepressants, are simply replacing one addiction with another. Whilst these may be helpful for an acute crisis, they should not be relied upon in the long term – major tranquillisers, for example, accelerate metabolic syndrome and all the complications that accompany it.

The brain is a remarkable computer. We are born with the hardware and the software is programmed through time and experience. Reprogramming of the brain, if considered necessary, would be a function of psychotherapy and counselling and this is beyond the scope of this book. However, any such therapies will be greatly enhanced by attention to diet, sleep, exercise, love, micronutrients, and hormonal and immunological interventions. Indeed, the power of these interventions is such that this may be all that is required. Throughout life, the brain creates a million new connections every second. This means that there is huge potential for healing and repair; it is simply a case of providing a good energy supply, the raw materials and the psychological direction to allow recovery.

What allows the brain to work quickly and efficiently is its energy supply. If this is impaired then the brain goes slow. Initially, the symptoms would be of 'foggy brain', by which I mean poor short-term memory, difficulty learning new things, poor mental stamina and concentration, difficulty multi-tasking and so on.

The energy molecule produced by mitochondria is ATP. This, along with DNA, is an evolutionarily ancient molecule which multitasks. ATP also

functions as a neurotransmitter – to be precise, a co-transmitter. Other neurotransmitters, such as serotonin, dopamine, GABA and acetylcholine, will not
work unless they are accompanied by a molecule of ATP. Improve ATP delivery and you improve all aspects of brain function. Improving ATP delivery is
a vital treatment for any brain dysfunction, from anxiety and premenstrual
tension to major psychosis and dementia. ATP is vital to power the electrical impulses that race along nerves and across synapses. A normal nerve will
pass a nerve impulse in 75 microseconds. The slower the time, the more we
'lose it'. Reaction times are slowed with alcohol. If this interval extends to 140
microseconds, one has dementia; longer than that and we go unconscious – as
exemplified by the effects of a general anaesthetic.

There is a further fascinating aspect – work by Nishihara (see note 5 page
231) suggests that microbes in the upper fermenting gut may appear in the brain
with the potential to ferment neurotransmitters into LSD-, amphetamine- and
ecstasy-like molecules. This could explain the hallucinations, paranoia and
irrational thoughts of psychosis and dementia. In this regard, treatment of the
fermenting gut may be useful – indeed, faecal bacteriotherapy has been used
in Parkinson's disease with good results.

Treatment of mental problems
- The Basic Package (see page 67).
- Tools to improve energy delivery systems (see page 90), especially a
  high-fat diet. Vitamin B12 by injection is especially helpful where there is
  low mood.
- Tools to treat the fermenting gut (see page 102).
- Psychotherapy to re-programme the brain – Hyper-vigilance is often hard-
  wired from a stressful childhood.

Cholesterol

As a nation we have been brainwashed into believing that a high-fat diet results
in high blood levels of cholesterol and that it is this that drives arteriosclerosis.
This does not stand up to scientific scrutiny. The situation is far more complex
and the following issues should be considered.

LDL cholesterol ('unfriendly') is associated with arteriosclerosis; for HDL
cholesterol ('friendly') the reverse is true. My patients eating Paleo-ketogenic
diets which are high in fat have high levels of HDL cholesterol. By contrast, the
carbohydrate addicts eating junk food diets have high levels of LDL cholesterol
and low levels of HDL.

Cholesterol is an essential part of the healing and repair of arteries damaged by blood pressure, inflammation, sugar and toxic stress. The critical factor is the proportion of good (HDL) to bad (LDL) cholesterol. High LDL and low HDL means that cholesterol is being actively employed in healing damaged arteries. It is therefore symptomatic of, and downstream of, active arterial repair. If there is repair, then there must also be ongoing damage.

Conversely, high HDL and low LDL suggests repair is not happening, ergo arteries are not being damaged.

High total cholesterol may be symptomatic of vitamin D deficiency or borderline hypothyroidism. Both are risk factors for arterial disease.

Statins lower levels of cholesterol, but the degree of lowering is not commensurate with their impact on arteriosclerosis. Biochemically, statins look like vitamin D and statin benefits arise from such. However, statins have a major biochemical glitch. They inhibit the body's own production of coenzyme Q10 – an essential molecule for energy production in mitochondria. This spells disaster for energy delivery systems, which are slowed, resulting in muscle problems, physical and mental fatigue and premature ageing. My CFS patients, who already have impaired mitochondria, do not tolerate statins.

Cholesterol is an essential molecule for membrane function, neurones and brain function. Low-fat, low-cholesterol diets are contributing to epidemics of dementia, CFS and organ failures.

Treatment of high cholesterol

- The Basic Package (see page 67).
- Measure vitamin D levels and check thyroid function.
- Do not suppress symptoms (that is, biochemical symptoms) with statins.

Constipation

Constipation is a clinical diagnosis – that is, based on symptoms and signs. A normal person on a good diet should open their bowels daily (on average) and effortlessly (no straining) to produce a large stool (oh dear, I've never weighed one!) – about 10–12 inches long, thick as a cucumber, soft, brown and fairly inoffensive.* Help is at hand with the Bristol Stool Chart so you can now grade 'em!

---

* **Historical note:** The 'Groom of the Stool' was one of the most high-ranking officials in the court of an English Monarch. His job was to be in charge of providing facilities for the Monarch's defecation and assisting in the cleansing. There is some evidence that the

Food should pass through the gut in 24–48 hours. You can easily measure your gut transit time by eating some beetroot (as the purple colouring goes straight through in many people) or sweetcorn, which is poorly digested. If food stays in the gut too long, it may be fermented to toxic substances and I suspect fermenting microbes are a risk factor for cancer. Constipation represents such a risk.

Treatment for constipation

- The Basic Package (see page 67).
- Allergy can certainly present with constipation and the commonest cause is cow's milk allergy. Apply the usual treatment package (see page 150).
- Prebiotics – Two-thirds of stool weight is bacteria. The majority are anaerobic fermenters – namely, bacteroides. There is no probiotic on the market which contains bacteroides but numbers can be increased by feeding with prebiotics. The best known of these are the fructo-oligosaccharides, which are naturally present in many plants, but others are present in artichokes, onion, brassicas, pulses, nuts and seeds. One can also take prebiotics as lactulose or, indeed, as fructo-oligosaccharides.
- Probiotics, such as kefir (1–3 cups daily) – These microbes will not survive in the gut but dead microbes still bulk up the stool.
- Water and minerals – Faeces contain a high proportion of water, and simple dehydration will remove water from faeces so that they become small, hard and difficult to pass. However, this cannot be corrected simply by drinking pure water. The reason for this, as explained in chapter 3, is that one cannot pee pure water; there are always minerals attached. So if one tries to re-hydrate just by drinking extra water without this being balanced by adequate minerals, either in the water or in the diet, this will result in further dehydration. Indeed, the worst mineral deficiencies I see occur in people who think it is healthy to drink several litres of water a day and in doing so wash out all their minerals. The body cannot put water into any one compartment; water actually follows minerals around. The biologists will understand that this is all about osmosis. One example of

---

'Groom' inspected the Monarch's stool and acted, de facto, as an early warning system for signs of illness. Eventually, this is where the term Privy Chamber is derived from to denote the Monarch's closest advisers. The position of the 'Groom' came to an end when Elizabeth I appointed, instead, the very first 'First Lady of the Bedchamber', Katherine Ashley. (Elizabeth was probably one of the first sugar addicts and her teeth went black through dental decay.)

this is how drinking water with too much mineral in it, such as sea water, also results in dehydration – the salt is peed out in the kidneys, but carries with it an awful lot more water than is contained in sea water. Drinking sea water causes massive dehydration and rapid death.

- Vitamin C to bowel tolerance – I recommend a single large dose of vitamin C at night to protect against infection and the upper fermenting gut. It also has a cathartic effect.
- Exercise – Exercise is a powerful stimulant to the gut and another reason to take a daily constitutional. Unfortunately, this is impossible for patients with CFS since this will make them worse and therefore they need to pay more attention to other factors.
- Hypothyroidism – Apply the usual treatment package (see page 95).
- Blockage – The gut can become blocked by strictures which can result after surgery, after inflammation (such as inflammatory bowel disease), or as a result of drug side effects. Aspirin-like drugs will cause severe bowel strictures in a minority of people.
- Drug side effects – Many medications are constipating because of their effect on the nerves which control gut movements. The commonest of these are the codeine-like analgesics, but many anticholinergic drugs, such as antidepressants, have a similar effect.

Diverticulosis

Diverticulosis is the long-term result of a lifetime of constipation. The small pouches that develop in the lining of the large bowel are unheard of except in the 'civilised', constipated modern Western cultures.

The large bowel is wrapped up in muscle: the circular muscle is continuous but the longitudinal muscle is in three strips. Between these strips there are areas of weakness and the pouches herniate out here. The hernias are called 'diverticula' (singular, 'diverticulum'). The trouble with these diverticula is that faecal material can get stuck in them, which may result in local bacterial overgrowth causing diverticulitis or 'left-sided appendicitis'. When infected during the very early stages, antibiotics may be helpful. However, pouches can rupture and cause peritonitis.

Treatment for diverticulosis

- As for constipation
- Tools to prevent infection – I give my patients who have already suffered one attack of diverticulitis, and so are at risk of further attacks, a course

of antibiotics to keep on hand and use at the first sign of symptoms. Diverticulitis is potentially dangerous and may result in gut perforation with peritonitis.

Osteoporosis

Osteoporosis is an inevitable result of modern Western diets and lifestyles which are high in sugar, refined carbohydrates and toxic stress, and deficient in micronutrients, sleep and exercise.

If vitamin D levels are good, then calcium, which is present in all living materials, will be well absorbed from the gut and, most importantly, laid down in bone. Calcium supplements over and above the Basic Package will not prevent osteoporosis. Neither will dairy products. Indeed, I could argue that dairy products make osteoporosis worse. We need calcium and magnesium in the proportion of 1:1 for good health. In dairy products it is in the proportion 10:1. Calcium and magnesium compete for absorption, so too much calcium results in a magnesium deficiency.

Strontium is of proven benefit in osteoporosis. It is a mineral which biochemically looks like calcium and is incorporated into bone instead of calcium, rendering bone tougher. Strontium is available on NHS prescription but unfortunately is made up with aspartame – something I would advise everyone to avoid because it is potentially neurotoxic.

Hormone replacement therapy has largely been abandoned as a prophylactic for osteoporosis because of its long-term risk of cancer. This was demonstrated by the Million Women Study[14] on HRT which had to be halted early because of excessive cancers in the hormone takers group.

Farmers, Gulf War veterans and pilots affected by aerotoxic syndrome are at increased risk of osteoporosis because of their exposures to organophosphate pesticides.

Warfarin (vitamin K antagonist) and proton-pump inhibitors (prevent mineral absorption) are risk factors for osteoporosis. Prescription bone builders like bisphosphonates often cause nausea and up to 5 per cent of people who take them risk osteonecrosis of the jaw.

Treatment of osteoporosis
- The Basic Package (see page 67).
- Exercise – It is rapidly changing gravitational fields within bone that create a piezo-electric effect and stimulate bone to be laid down. It may be that rebounding (exercise on a mini-trampoline) is an efficient way to achieve this.

- Extra nutritional supplements:

  Vitamin D – This must be in the form of vitamin D3, up to 10,000 IU daily or whatever is needed to achieve a blood level between 75 and 200 nmol/l. The best source of vitamin D is sunshine.

  Strontium – 250–500 mg of elemental strontium daily.

  Pregnenolone, 10–25 mg sublingually daily. DHEA is an essential hormone for normal bone density. Levels fall with age. It is, as I call it, an 'acquired metabolic dyslexia'.

  Vitamin K, 10 mg daily – This is essential for normal bone formation. Warfarin, for example, is a vitamin K blocker and a risk factor for osteoporosis.

  Hypochlorhydria is a major risk factor since we need an acid stomach to absorb minerals and strontium.

- Check thyroid function – Both under- and over-active thyroid are risk factors for osteoporosis.
- Tools to treat mechanical problems: structure, friction and wear and tear (see page 111).
- Do not use HRT – The Million Women Study on HRT had to be abandoned early because those women taking HRT had increased cancer rates.

I have collected bone-density scans of 14 patients before and after a tailored package of the above interventions. In every case, where the regime has been complied with, bone density has either remained the same or improved. Although the figures are small, the statistics are powerful. And once again I employ the logic of Ovid: 'The result validates the deeds.'

Eye disease: macular degeneration, glaucoma, cataracts

Weight for weight, the retina consumes energy 10 times faster than the brain. The energy demands are so high because the business of converting a light signal to an electrical signal that the brain can read requires it. Energy production is never totally efficient – exhaust gases in the form of free radicals are produced which damage the eye, more so where there is poor antioxidant status.

Treatment for eye disease

- The Basic Package (see page 67).
- Tools to correct antioxidant status.

III. Conditions driven by the long-term effects of metabolic syndrome and inflammation

Heart disease

Heart disease is an inevitable long-term outcome of metabolic syndrome. Because the heart is greatly demanding of energy, it is one of the first organs to be affected by arteriosclerosis and poor energy delivery systems (mitochondrial, thyroid and adrenal function). Modern medicine has become wonderfully skilled at techniques to identify and bypass arterial narrowings with stents and bypasses, drugs to control angina and pacemakers to correct rhythm disturbances. However, in doing so, the underlying threads that result in heart disease are often lost. Those threads are:

- **Arteriosclerosis** – See page 135 for treatment.
- **Poor energy delivery systems,** notably poor mitochondrial function. This I learned about from the cardiologist Dr Stephen Sinatra, whose book *The Sinatra Solution* makes essential reading for anyone with heart disease. He describes many cases of heart failure and dysrhythmias resolving simply through nutritional supplements to support mitochondria. Cardiac muscle is made up 25 per cent by weight of mitochondria. These are the vital engines that take fuel from the bloodstream and burn it in the presence of oxygen to make energy for the heart to beat powerfully as a pump. If this energy delivery mechanism fails, there is a switch into anaerobic metabolism with the production of lactic acid. Lactic-acid burn in the heart results in the symptom of angina. If the heart beats weakly, then cardiac output will fall and ultimately this results in heart failure. This is called cardiomyopathy. This is common in my CFS/ME patients where there is poor mitochondrial function, so when energy demand exceeds delivery there is a switch into anaerobic metabolism, with the production of lactic acid. Lactic acid causes angina. If blood supply is reasonable, then, with rest, lactic acid will quickly (within a minute or two) convert back to glucose via the Cori cycle. In anaerobic metabolism, one molecule of glucose generates only two molecules of ATP and, of course, lactic acid. However, to shunt lactic acid back to glucose requires six molecules of ATP (this takes time – several minutes, possibly hours), so the lactic acid angina pain is much more prolonged where mitochondrial function is impaired, as in CFS/ME.

The symptoms of chronic (by which I mean long-standing) heart failure arise for the following reasons:

i. Blood and fluids are not efficiently cleared and a backlog forms:
- lungs – pulmonary oedema with cough, shortness of breath and susceptibility to infections
- legs – pitting oedema; possibly ulcers
- gut – loss of appetite, poor digestion

ii. All organs are starved of fuel and oxygen, which eventually results in organ failure, for example:
- brain – therefore acute confusion or dementia develop
- kidneys – kidney failure results
- bone marrow – anaemia develops
- body – CFS

iii. The heart dilates, so the valves no longer 'fit', especially the mitral valve. Some blood leaks back, making heart beats increasingly inefficient.

The above mechanisms result in a downward spiral of malfunction and so heart failure has a poor prognosis, with most sufferers dying within five years of diagnosis. The following contribute:

- **Poor electrical function of pacemaker** – The heart must beat in a coordinated way – too slow will reduce cardiac output; too fast means the heart may not have time to fill and again cardiac output will fall. A mixture, such as with the irregular pulse of atrial fibrillation, will reduce cardiac output by 20 per cent.
- **Poisoning** – Pacemaker problems may derive from poor energy delivery to the pacemaker (see above), which could result from poisoning. We are currently seeing epidemics of tachydysrhythmias, such as ventricular ectopics (extra heartbeats that are not initiated by the pacemaker) and atrial fibrillation. I learned this first when I helped 23 farmers with sheep-dip poisoning in a group action against the manufacturers of sheep dip. The average age of these farmers was well below 50, but 15 of the 23 had been diagnosed with significant cardiac dysrhythmias from ventricular ectopics, paroxysmal atrial tachycardia, paroxysmal atrial fibrillation, atrial fibrillation, etc. In this case, the poisoning clearly arose from organophosphate pesticides. (Sadly we were unable to see this action to a conclusion because of lack of funds.)

- **Heavy metals** – These bio-accumulate in the heart and may also disrupt electrical conduction; importantly, chelation therapy is of proven benefit.

In the early stages of pacemaker disease, often the problem is intermittent. It may start with occasional ventricular ectopics – these should be seen as early warning symptoms. Often doctors dismiss ventricular ectopics as nothing to worry about, but this is a golden opportunity to tackle the cause. In these early stages, the pacemaker is irritable and can be fired up into misdemeanours by caffeine or adrenaline – often drugs to block such are prescribed, for example, beta blockers. Patients are advised to reduce stress (adrenaline). But we need adrenaline to have fun! Well, I do. Beta blockers take the fun out of life, increase the risk of diabetes and reduce the ability to get fit.

Treatment of heart disease
- As for arteriosclerosis (see page 135) – By the time heart disease is manifest, there may be serious arterial disease and surgical techniques may be essential to bypass narrowings.
- Tools to address energy delivery mechanisms – That is, mitochondrial function (coenzyme Q10, 250–500 mg; acetyl-l-carnitine, 1–2 grams; D-ribose, 5–15 grams; niacinamide [NAD] 1,500 mg slow release; extra magnesium, possibly intravenously), thyroid function and adrenal function.
- Tools to address toxic stress, such as toxic metals by urine analysis after taking the chelating agent DMSA. Consider fat biopsy to look for pesticide residues or volatile organic compounds. Use detox regimes (see page 105), appropriate to the toxin, but most often the problem is toxic metals.
- Tools to address inflammation.
- Identify any clotting tendency, over and above the clotting tendency of metabolic syndrome, such as taking the Pill or HRT, antiphospholipid syndrome, Leiden V (a genetically inherited disorder of blood clotting) and so on.

Heart attack
'Heart attack' is a descriptive term which does not tell us the underlying mechanisms that lead to it. Symptoms arise because the blood supply is reduced or cut off, so energy delivery halts. Within a few seconds there is a switch into anaerobic metabolism with the production of lactic acid. This lactic acid burn is angina. It is very painful, increasingly so as levels of lactic acid rise. If uncorrected there will be muscle death with myocardial infarction. The pain of a myocardial infarction is one of the most severe one can suffer.

Energy delivery may be reduced because the artery is narrowed by blocks (arteriosclerosis, with plaque rupture) or arterial muscle spasm (adrenaline from shock, panic or stress). Energy delivery may be reduced because of a low cardiac output state, such as the heart being in a dysrhythmia (see page 198), because of an acute valve lesion (e.g. mitral incompetence, aortic incompetence) or because of poor mitochondrial function. Often there is a combination of factors.

Immediate treatment for heart attack

This will involve urgent hospital admission for diagnosis of the cause of the heart attack, possibly clot-busting treatments, drugs to control dysrhythmias, drugs to control pain, oxygen and so on.

Longer-term treatment for heart attack

This should be as for heart disease.

Stroke

A stroke is a neurological deficit that results when the energy delivery to a part of the brain is so poor that there is insufficient power for neurones to work. The vast majority of strokes result from arterial disease. Altogether, 85 per cent are thromboembolic – that is, caused by a blood clot from arterial disease or from formation in the lining of the heart when there is a dysrhythmia, typically atrial fibrillation, the other 15 per cent of strokes result from bleeds into the brain. An acute stroke requires urgent attention at a specialist centre to determine whether it has resulted from a bleed or a block because, in the latter case, clot-busting drugs are essential. Some people are fortunate to just experience a 'TIA', or mini temporary stroke. This should flag up an urgent need to put in place all the interventions to prevent further episodes.

Treatment of strokes caused by thrombosis

- Treatment of arteriosclerosis (see page 135)
- Treatment of dysrhythmias, such as atrial fibrillation (see page 198)
- Identify any clotting tendency, in addition to the clotting tendency of metabolic syndrome, such as taking the Pill or HRT, autoimmune issues (such as anti-phospholipid syndrome) or genetic problems (such as Leiden V). Any inflammatory process makes blood sticky.
- Identify allergies – Migraine can be associated with TIA – that is, so-called hemiplegic migraine.

Cancer

Also see chapters 2 and 3, on growth promotion (page 60) and tools of the trade to treat (page 113).

Treatment of cancer

Treatment of cancer is a numbers game. It is all about starving the little wretches (cancerous cells) out and killing them at the same time. The conventional medical approach is to surgically remove or kill cancer cells, whereas nutritional therapies starve them out and improve immune function. There is a happy synergism between the two to provide the best chance of survival.

Interventions that may be additionally helpful in specific cancers include:

- **Skin cancer** (other than melanoma) – at the first sign of sun damage to skin I recommend Curaderm, which is extract of eggplant. It is highly effective in treating solar keratosis, early basal cell carcinoma (rodent ulcers) and early squamous cell carcinomas. If there is no sign of remission after eight weeks of use, then consultant opinion is necessary. (This treatment is ineffective for melanoma, for which urgent consultant opinion is always required.)
- **Prostate cancer** – Professor Ben Pfeiffer has a regime of supplements which is effective. See www.canceractive.com/cancer-active-page -link.aspx?n=1631.

See my website (www.drmyhill.com) for more as I learn more.

Treatment of degenerative neurological conditions: Parkinson's disease (PD), Alzheimer's disease and Creutzfeldt-Jakob's disease

Note: Motor neurone disease may also be a prion disorder.

We are seeing epidemics of these neurodegenerative conditions, which are a further inevitable long-term consequence of metabolic syndrome. Alzheimer's disease, for example, has been dubbed 'type III diabetes of the brain' (although this is a misnomer – the actual pathology of this type of dementia is atherosclerotic; true Alzheimer's is a prion disorder).

The problem with prion disorders is a similar problem to cancer. A pathological process has been switched on which then has a momentum of its own – indeed, I think of prion disorders as protein cancers. Stopping the smoker from smoking does not cure his lung cancer – it is too late. Current figures are that 50 per cent of people over the age of 80 will suffer dementia. Meanwhile, I am now seeing Parkinson's disease in people in their early 40s. By the time the clinical picture arises it is too late for curative treatment.

The aim should be to slow down the progression of the disease, hopefully to an extent where healing and repair exceed damage. There has to be a reason why Stephen Hawking has survived motor neurone disease for 30 years when for most the prognosis is much worse.*

Treatment of prion disorders

- The Basic Package (see page 67)
- Tools to improve energy delivery systems: mitochondria, thyroid and adrenal function. The brain is largely made up of fats. It is enormously demanding of energy and it needs fats to deliver energy as well as requiring fats as a fuel source. Indeed, the myelin sheaths which are wrapped around axons have adopted mitochondrial biochemistry so as to deliver energy to nerve cell axons. Our present infatuation with low-fat diets, low cholesterol and statins are fuelling the current epidemic of degenerative brain disorders. A high-fat diet is a vital part of improving brain function.
- Tools for detoxification – could be a heavy metal (measure urine toxic elements following a chelating agent) or a pesticide (fat biopsy) and do appropriate detox regimes.
- Tools to treat inflammation – I use vitamin B12 by injection as a routine with almost any neurological disorder.
- Tools to treat autoimmunity – there appear to be two stages in prion disorders – firstly a slow build-up of prion protein which behaves like a rotten apple to twist adjacent proteins so they are rendered indestructible and cannot be broken down by the body. These prions gradually build up and interfere with normal cell metabolism. Then there is a second stage when the immune system suddenly recognises that this build-up of prion is abnormal and this triggers an inflammatory response. This is not curative because prion is such a tough molecule. The ongoing inflammation results in an escalation of damage.

---

* **Historical note:** Stephen Hawking took a first in Natural Sciences at Oxford University before obtaining a PhD at the University of Cambridge, where he was instated as the 17th Lucasian Professor of Mathematics. Sir Isaac Newton was the 2nd such Professor and the current holder is Michael Cates, a British physicist. Some of Hawking's colleagues attribute the way in which he has adapted his working style, as a result of his illness, and his ability to visualise solutions to problems, as having had an impact on his research and his view of the Universe.

- Stem cell therapy – I think this is where the future lies for established prion disorders. Stem cells have a remarkable ability to differentiate into any cell, depending on its 3D position within the body. So injecting stem cells into the substantia nigra of the brain should be a logical treatment for Parkinson's. I currently advise my patients to do all the above but keep looking out for stem cell therapy advances.

Gynaecological problems: polycystic ovarian syndrome (PCOS), endometriosis, irregular periods, low libido, menorrhagia, infertility

The selfish gene theories of Richard Dawkins (*The Selfish Gene*, 1976) tell us that the only function of life is to procreate. These ideas were taken further in *The Extended Phenotype* (1982), where Dawkins notes that natural selection is:

> *the process whereby replicators out-propagate each other.*

Dawkins is currently an emeritus fellow of New College, Oxford, and was Oxford University's Professor for Public Understanding of Science from 1995 until 2008.

However, the business of procreation is greatly demanding of energy and raw materials. The commonest cause of infertility – outside the problems contemporary Westerners have – is starvation. In Westerners, calories are in abundance. For them (us), the problem is a combination of micronutrient deficiency, toxic stress and upper fermenting gut – that is to say, the same causes as for metabolic syndrome. Address metabolic syndrome thoroughly with the Basic Package and many problems will be resolved.

The most sensitive test of nutritional status in women of child-bearing age is a regular and trouble-free menstrual cycle.

Most importantly, avoid using sex hormones, such as the Pill or HRT, to impose a regular cycle. This is symptom suppression. These hormones drive metabolic syndrome (and all its complications) and are carcinogenic growth-promoters. The same is true of fertility-enhancing drugs.

Treatment of gynaecological disorders

- The Basic Package (see page 67).
- Investigate and treat sexually transmitted disease – Many STDs are sub-clinical, with no overt symptoms; these must be identified and eradicated.

- Identify and treat toxic load – Use tools for detoxification (see page 33).
- Employ tools for improving energy delivery – The business of procreation demands energy.

IV. Conditions associated with inflammation

Autoimmunity – the general approach to treatment

The immune system has a difficult job to do. It has to recognise those things which are safe and allow them to enter the body, where they help us survive. This, of course, is what digestion and absorption of foods is all about. Indeed, 90 per cent of the immune system is gut associated. It also has to decide what is dangerous to the body, such as infection with bacteria, viruses, yeasts or parasites. Having established that there is a threat, it then has to determine the level of reaction against it – in other words, just the right amount of inflammation to control that threat because too much will damage the body.

The immune reactions that we see in infection we also see in allergy, autoimmunity and conditions associated with inflammation.

We know that much autoimmunity is driven by infection with microbes – most commonly viruses, but bacteria, yeast, parasites and vaccination are also implicated. Not everyone develops autoimmunity – there may be a genetic susceptibility. Furthermore, where there are pro-inflammatory forces the chances of developing autoimmunity are greater. The same principles are likely to be true for allergy.

Problems arise when the immune system gets its wires crossed and starts to react against things which it should not. When it reacts, it produces inflammation and it is this that gives us symptoms. Autoimmunity is all about allergy to our own body material – it is a completely useless reaction and, of course, destructive. So it is with allergy, also.

One can sensitise to anything under the sun (including the sun!) – for example, to foods, biological inhalants, chemicals, micro-organisms from the outside world (viruses, bacteria, yeasts, parasites, etc) and micro-organisms from the fermenting gut (bacteria, yeasts, parasites and possibly viruses).

Treatment of allergy and autoimmunity – the general approach

- The Basic Package (see page 67)
- Employ the tools to treat inflammatory conditions (see page 66)
- Identify and avoid provoking foods (food allergy tests are not reliable)
- Identify and avoid provoking biological inhalant allergens (skin tests and RAST tests can be helpful but false negatives are common) – Biological

allergens are water soluble and so a shower and change of clothes are often helpful to reduce exposure

- Identify and avoid provoking chemicals (lymphocyte sensitivity tests can be helpful)
- Identify and avoid provoking electromagnetic radiation
- Use desensitising techniques such as EPD, neutralisation, oral immuno-therapy or homeopathy (see page 66)

You will notice that avoidance is a large part of the treatment package and, once again, like prevention, this is often better than 'cure'.

I do prescribe medications – such as cromoglycate, antihistamines and, possibly, steroids – to make life comfortable and damp down useless inflammations which may develop a momentum of their own.

There is now good evidence to show that the presence of auto-antibodies is a strong predictor of disease and so treatment should start before clinical symptoms arise. However, I know of no method that will switch off auto-immunity. Like prion disorders and cancer, they are switched on by modern Western diets and lifestyles, but we do not know how to switch them off. Since autoimmunity now affects 1 in 20 Westerners, and allergy about 1 in 3, prevention is vital. However, we may be able to identify factors that drive autoimmunity, such as chronic infection, and so treat.

Anaphylaxis

Anaphylaxis is a major allergic reaction with the potential to kill. It should always be taken seriously. It can be caused by any substance, but the commonest reactions follow ingestion of foods, stings from wasps and bees, and exposures to chemicals. It is not uncommon to see anaphylactic reactions with exercise, and up to 50 per cent of these are associated with foods.

Treatment for anaphylaxis

- **Mild reactions** – Itchy skin; flushed skin; blotchy skin; a raised, red, itchy rash; swelling of the mouth; tickling, tingling or itching of the throat, mouth and lips; stomach ache. Take antihistamines – any type will do. Crunch up in the mouth and swallow. Apply cold water or ice packs to the affected area – sometimes this is sufficient to stop the reaction progressing. If the symptoms do not settle, and if available, nebulise an ampoule of adrenaline. If the above symptoms progress, or there is any hint of further reactions, do not waste time. Use injected adrenaline or EpiPen if available AND get to hospital.

- **Severe/anaphylactic reactions** – Marked swelling of the lips or tongue, difficulty in swallowing, wheeze or difficulty in breathing, change in voice or inability to speak, drowsiness, blue lips, feeling faint, loss of consciousness, abnormal pulse – it may be going fast, or conversely might be going very slow; blood pressure may fall. If in doubt as to whether or not to use an EpiPen or adrenaline by injection, use it. No one has ever died following an intramuscular injection of adrenaline. The injection needs to be into the muscle.

Some people need a second injection of EpiPen, and so make sure you always have two to hand. Any anaphylactic or near- anaphylactic reaction must be seen and assessed by a doctor urgently. If adrenaline is needed, also take prednisolone 30 mg (6 tablets) or hydrocortisone 100 mg. These take up to six hours to work but they help to prevent a second attack.

There is a very useful website called LIFELINE, www.jext.co.uk. They can send you a dummy EpiPen for you to practise with. Adrenaline has a short lifespan, so do check the dates on your ampoules and EpiPen regularly. I like all my patients to have three EpiPens – one for the house, one for the car and one for the handbag (or 'manbag', as appropriate).

Asthma, chronic obstructive airway's disease (COAD/COPD), rhinitis, sinusitis, ENT problems

Asthma and rhinitis are too often diagnosed as deficiencies of blue and brown inhalers and treated accordingly. Scant attention is paid to causation.

Treatment for respiratory disorders

- Treat allergy or autoimmunity: see the general approach (page 150); foods and gut bacteria are often overlooked as allergens.
- Address dairy allergy, which often results in mucus production with catarrhal symptoms. These include chronic rhinitis, recurrent tonsillitis, glue ears, eustachian tube dysfunction and sore throats.
- Consider moulds as a potential cause – Moulds in the environment are a major cause of asthma, especially in damp housing or mouldy hay and straw for livestock. When combined with recurrent courses of antibiotics together with high-carbohydrate diets, mould and yeast infections of the lungs ensue and may be over-looked as a cause of ongoing disease.
- EPD (see page 199) works well where avoidance is not possible.

- Environmental pollution is a major cause of asthma and COAD/COPD – This may be from in the house (sick building syndrome) or from outside. Sufferers may be allergic to pollutants, but POPs may drive inflammation directly. The work of the late Dr Dick van Steenis[15] highlighted the effects of polluting industry by looking at the use of asthma inhalers in school children living around or downwind of polluting industry (power, chemical and manufacturing). In the areas studied, up to 20 per cent of children were using inhalers compared with 1 per cent of those living in unpolluted zones.
- Salt pipes are often helpful. (The mechanism of action is uncertain but asthma is rare in people working in the salt-mining industry.)
- Hyperventilation is common with asthma, and sometimes rhinitis – Learning to sing or play a wind instrument is often helpful. So is the Buteyko breathing training method, which is of proven benefit in treating hyperventilation.
- Magnesium by nebuliser or intravenous injection is effective in treating an acute attack.

With severe brittle asthma, always have bronchodilators (ideally by nebuliser), steroids and antibiotics available, know how to use them and do not be afraid of using them.

Eczema and urticaria

Eczema and urticaria are inflammations of the skin. Inflammation may have many causes and since the skin is the interface between the outside world and the inside body, there are many possible causes of this inflammation.

Treatment for eczema and urticaria
- Treat allergy or autoimmunity: see the general approach (page 150)
- Increase the barrier between the outside and inside world by:
  Avoiding soap and water, which remove oils from the skin. Use coconut oil to restore oils – it feeds the friendly skin bacteria which displace unfriendly microbes.
  Reducing staphylococci on the skin – We all have bacteria on our skin but eczema patients sensitise to these bacteria, especially staphylococci. These bacteria inhabit the cracks in the skin where there is an allergic/infectious reaction, causing inflammation and itching. I think this explains why children are prone to eczema in the creases

of the elbows and behind the knees where the skin is thinner. I recommend using antibacterial ointments (no sensitising preservatives), such as fucidin ointment, applied liberally to any broken or cracked skin. Sunshine and salt water reduce microbial numbers so a seaside holiday is often helpful.

Reducing house dust mite exposure – Many eczema sufferers are house dust mite sensitive and sufferers should take anti-house–dust mite measures. Allergy to animal furs can be tested by rubbing the offending fur into the skin to see if there is a reaction, such as itching or redness.

Paying attention to chemical sensitivity/pro-inflammatory irritant effects – Washing powders and rinsing agents are markedly sensitising. Just because it has been used for years does not mean one cannot sensitise. Chlorine in water is very sensitising and many eczema sufferers do not tolerate public swimming baths. Some children do not tolerate the chlorine in tap water. Recently, chloramine has been used in drinking water rather than chlorine, and this is toxic and allergenic. ACE inhibitors are good at triggering urticaria. Synthetic fabrics are often irritating to a sensitive skin – use cotton. Take care with cosmetics.

• Try nutritional interventions such as:

Consuming high doses of omega-6 and omega-3 essential fatty acids – Indeed, a preparation called Epogam used to be on NHS prescription specifically for the treatment of eczema. I suggest a tablespoon of hemp oil.

Taking zinc supplements – This is a common deficiency in people with allergies and 20 mg daily should be taken in addition to the nutritional supplements I advise people to take at all times (see page 72).

Identify and avoid allergies to foods – Any food can cause eczema or urticaria, but in my experience those most commonly implicated are dairy products, egg, additives, colourings, flavourings, gluten grains and, in the case of urticaria, salicylates (for example, citrus fruits, berries, tomatoes). If a baby develops eczema and is breast-fed, then the mother must avoid the provoking food since food antigens are readily able to pass from the maternal gut into the blood stream and from there into the breast milk. The mother needs to eat a Paleo-ketogenic diet. Mothers who consume probiotics during pregnancy and breast feeding protect their babies from allergic problems.

Identifying and addressing upper fermenting gut – I suspect this
is a cause of eczema and urticaria because of allergic reactions to
microbes. In particular, I suspect varicose eczema is a symptom of
allergy to gut microbes.

Desensitisation: Eczema and urticaria patients often have multiple causes
for their skin problems and therefore I have a low threshold for starting desensitisation. I like to use enzyme potentiated desensitisation (EPD – see page
199), which I find particularly effective in treating eczema. Indeed, if somebody told me I had to save EPD for just one group of patients, then it would
be for eczema since the results are reliably good.

Psoriasis

I know of no single formula that works in all cases of psoriasis. Yeasts are often
a player, possibly because of allergy, so I would start with an anti-yeast regime.
Most importantly with psoriasis, don't use steroids. They will temporarily
damp down the problem, but when the steroids are stopped psoriasis will flare;
in addition, in high doses they thin the skin.

Treatment for psoriasis
- The Basic Package (see page 67)
- Employ the tools to treat the fermenting gut (see page 102) – start with
  yeast by excluding from the diet yeast and all sugars, including fruit sugars
- Employ the tools to treat inflammation (see page 66)
- Sunshine is excellent for acne and psoriasis; indeed, high-dose UV light is
  often used to treat severe psoriasis
- Vitamin D-based creams, such as calcipotriol, may help

Acne and rosacea

Acne is driven by male sex hormones (present in both sexes from the
menarche [start of menstruation] onwards). In the early stages the skin pro-
ducess excess keratin, which blocks the cysts at the base of hairs; later these
become inflamed and infected by propionic-bacteria. This has markedly pro-
inflammatory effects which I can only think are allergy driven. It explains why
acne responds well to antibiotics because they reduce this infectious/allergic
drive. I suspect the allergic/inflammatory drive in rosacea is largely from the
upper fermenting gut.

Acne can be a detox reaction – The first description of this was chloracne, associated with organochlorine poisoning. The skin cannot tell if chemicals are on the way in or out, and so a similar reaction may ensue with detoxification in the sauna. Some people develop acne with B12 injections and again I suspect this is a detox reaction as chemicals are mobilised.

Treatment of acne and rosacea

- The Basic Package (page 67) – Dairy allergy commonly results in zits (as my daughters like to call them: the word 'zit' is one of those fascinating words of unknown origin; it is thought to have entered common usage around the mid 1960s among American teenagers; the only slightly plausible explanation for its origin is from the German 'Zitze', meaning teat or nipple).
- Take additional nutritional supplements:
  Zinc 20 mg daily.
  Pantothenic acid (vitamin B5) – There are many studies demonstrating benefit. High doses of up to 10 grams daily need to be used (the highest strength I can find is 500 mg so 20 tablets a day may be needed).
    B5 is extremely safe, with no known side effects and no toxicity.
- Use the tools to treat inflammation (see page 66).
- Reduce microbial contamination of the skin – Coconut oil works well. I use an antiseptic spray containing colloidal silver, zinc and vitamin C.
- Sunshine and salt water – A beach holiday is often excellent for clearing acne.
- Ultraviolet light is helpful (remember to protect the eyes).
- Treat the upper fermenting gut (see page 102).
- Antibiotics – Again, these undoubtedly work. Part of the reason is that they kill bacteria on the skin, but part of the effect may be that they treat the upper fermenting gut. My guess is that this is more of a problem in rosacea.

Note: do not use roaccutane. This drug is isotretinoin, metabolised in the body to tretinoin, which is used for cancer chemotherapy. It permanently destroys 'moisture producing' cells on organ surfaces and may lead to permanently dry skin, eyes, mouth, etc. It also has profound effects on the brain. I have seen several patients with severe long-term ill health as a result of this drug.

Note: do not use the Pill. It does not address the underlying causes and has serious side effects. It is effective but encourages metabolic syndrome and is growth promoting (see page 60).

Irritable bowel syndrome, GERD, upper gut ulcers*

These symptoms are almost always caused by a combination of food allergy, fermenting gut and poor digestion. It is essential to identify the underlying mechanisms that result in these clinical pictures because this has obvious implications for management. Conventional medicine often prescribes symptom-suppressing drugs, which tend to worsen gut function, with the potential to make the underlying problem worse or induce other problems. A particular hate of mine are the proton-pump inhibitors ('PPI', such as Omeprazole), which result in hypochlorhydria. An acid stomach is a vital defence against infection, essential for digesting protein (otherwise large, antigenically interesting molecules present downstream with the potential to switch on allergy), preventing upper gut fermentation and allowing the absorption of minerals. PPIs are a risk factor for stomach cancer, oesophageal cancer and osteoporosis.

Treatment of bowel problems

- The Basic Package (see page 67).
- Treat allergy or autoimmunity: see the general approach, page 150.
- Employ the tools to treat the fermenting gut (see page 102) – These could include targeting *Helicobacter pylori* for GERD and ulcers, and yeast, bacterial overgrowths or gut parasites. Improving gut function may resolve the allergies, so I would not start on desensitisation until poor digestion and fermenting issues have been addressed.
- Employ the tools to treat inflammation (see page 66).

Migraine and headaches†

Treatment of migraine and headaches

- Use the Basic Package (see page 67) – This, done well, will prevent the vast majority of headaches.
- Employ the tools to address energy delivery (see page 90) – Intravenous magnesium is highly effective in the treatment of acute migraine.
- Employ the tools to treat inflammation.

---

* Gastro-oesphageal reflux disease

† **Historical Note:** An early description of migraines is contained within the Ebers papyrus, dated from around 1500 BC. In 200 BC, writings from the Hippocratic School of Medicine described the visual auras which precede the headache in some sufferers. Galen of Pergamon used the term 'hemicrania' (half-head), from which the word migraine was eventually derived.

Inflammatory bowel disease:
Crohn's disease, ulcerative colitis

In treating these conditions, conventional medicine pays scant regard to causation but relies on symptom-suppressing medication. This is not best practice because both Crohn's and ulcerative colitis are potentially life-threatening conditions that respond well when underlying mechanisms are identified and corrected. Allergy to foods is a major player, and in ulcerative colitis probably allergy to gut flora. Inflammatory bowel disease (IBD) often has an arthritis associated with it, possibly as the allergic reaction to bacteria in the gut results in joint symptoms. The mechanism may be molecular mimicry, as described by Dr Alan Ebringer.[16] The idea here is that the body makes antibodies against gut bacteria, which then cross-react with the self to cause back pain and typically early morning stiffness.

Treatment of inflammatory bowel disease

- The Basic Package (see page 67) – In Crohn's disease almost always there is allergy; this was shown by Dr John Hunter at Addenbrooke's Hospital, Cambridge – patients responded as well to an elimination diet as to drug medication including steroids. Nearly all are intolerant of grains. By contrast with ulcerative colitis where there are often multiple allergens, in Crohn's disease usually just a few foods are implicated.
- Use the tools to treat inflammation (page 66) – In an unpublished study by Dr McEwen, EPD (see page 199) was effective in reducing both reliance on medication and the number of relapses.
- Employ the tools to treat the upper fermenting gut (see page 102) – The probiotic *Lactobacillus plantarum* is markedly anti-inflammatory and present in the NHS prescribable probiotic VSL 3.
- Try faecal bacteriotherapy (see page 105) – This therapy is highly effective in ulcerative colitis, with one course of treatment resulting in long, possibly permanent, remission.
- Treat *Mycobacterium avium* subspecies para-tuberculosis infection – Work by Professor John Hermon-Taylor at St George's Hospital, London has demonstrated that some early cases of Crohn's can be completely cured by antibiotics.[17] He has shown the presence of a tuberculosis-like organism called *Mycobacterium avium* subspecies para-tuberculosis, present in the gut of Crohn's patients. This is the same bacterium that causes Johne's disease in cattle and is thought to be acquired by humans through drinking milk. The pasteurisation of milk does not kill this bacterium,

which Professor Hermon-Taylor has shown to be present in about 10 per cent of all milk samples. We are all exposed to this bacterium, but not all of us become infected. On his death bed Pasteur famously said, 'It's the terrain, not the germ.'

- Worms – These have a useful anti-inflammatory effect on the gut. Indeed, this illustrates the 'hygiene hypothesis'. The immune system needs exposure to bacteria and parasites for it to be correctly programmed. Modern worm-free life means the gut no longer obtains this essential programming and the immune system starts to react inappropriately.

Irritable bladder syndrome, interstitial cystitis

Any part of the body can react allergically. Irritable bladder syndrome is the equivalent of irritable bowel syndrome, but affecting the bladder rather than the bowel, and can be caused by allergies to foods, micro-organisms or chemicals. However, the commonest problem is allergy to yeast or bacteria that spill over from the upper fermenting gut. Interstitial cystitis is a painful chronic bladder inflammation which I suspect starts with allergic bladder. The symptoms of the allergic bladder are exactly the same as those of bladder infection – that is, a constant desire to pee (stranguary), increased frequency of peeing, pain on peeing (cystitis) and, possibly, passing blood.

The difference between allergy and infection is the number of organisms present. Infected bladder is defined by the presence of more than 10,000 bacteria per millilitre of urine. This can be measured as part of microscopy and culture on a urine sample. It can also be diagnosed using Multistix. This is an extremely useful DIY test because one can very quickly tell from the simple dip test if the urine contains abnormal amounts of white cells, nitrites, red blood cells, protein, sugar, ketones and so on. It is a very sensitive test and often sufferers are told that they do have an infection on dipstick, but microscopy and culture are normal and therefore there is no infection!

If symptoms improve with antibiotics but urine cultures are negative, this suggests bacterial allergy. If antibiotics make the symptoms worse, then this could point to yeast sensitivity. If antifungals improve the symptoms, then this could point to yeast allergy. Yeast and bacteria are normally present in the gut and they are normally present in our food.

Treatment of irritable bladder

- The Basic Package (see page 67).
- Treat upper fermenting gut (see page 102).

- Prevent bacteria from sticking to the lining of the urinary tract:
  D-mannose is specific for *E. coli*, the commonest cause of urinary tract infection and allergy. *E. coli* sticks to the lining by a sugar receptor; saturate this with D-mannose and *E. coli* passes through, causing no problems at all!
  Bicarbonate is a traditional remedy for cystitis and my guess is that it works by again interfering with adherence to the bladder lining. I suggest potassium citrate or magnesium carbonate to alkalinise the urine.

Joint, connective tissue and muscle problems

There seems to be a general acceptance that joint and muscle pain is an inevitable part of ageing. This is not so – but it is an almost inevitable part of metabolic syndrome. Worse, the front-line, doctor-recommended remedies are symptom-suppressing pain killers and anti-inflammatory drugs. Using these would be expected to accelerate the problem since these drugs allow a patient to use a joint that actually needs resting. Furthermore, inflammation is an essential part of the healing and repair process. Indeed, non-steroidal anti-inflammatories (NSAIs) have been shown to accelerate the rate of degeneration of cartilage and joints.

The cardinal symptom of degenerative joint, connective tissue and muscle problems is that exercise makes things worse and rest improves them. Interestingly, where there is an inflammatory component the pain and stiffness are worse in the morning. This may be because healing and repair occur at night, or because of allergy withdrawal symptoms.

A diagnosis I am increasingly recognising is where allergy affects muscles. Because muscles can only react in one way – through contraction – this produces symptoms such as cramp, acute stiff neck, restless legs, jerking muscles, twitching muscles and 'fasciculation'. I suspect some muscle dystonia reactions may be driven by allergy also.

Allergic muscles

Diagnosing allergic muscles may be difficult because reactions are often delayed. They may start 24 or 48 hours after allergen exposure and last for several days. Often there is acute lancinating pain. This pain may be so severe that the sufferer literally collapses. Typically this lasts a few seconds or minutes and the sufferer looks like he (or maybe even she!) is a right old hypochondriac.

Pain is triggered by stretching the affected muscle. Initially, any stretch will cause it; then, as things settle down, only a sudden stretch will do so. The sufferer protects himself from the pain by moving slowly. Clinically, this is described as stiffness. Other muscles in the vicinity of the allergic muscles may also go into spasm to protect against sudden inadvertent stretching, and this causes a more generalised muscle spasm and stiffness. There is further complication because if muscles contract inappropriately they can damage themselves, literally by pulling themselves apart. Further pain develops because the blood circulation through muscle is disturbed and there is the build-up of metabolites, in particular lactic acid. Lactic acid causes pain. So often we then see a particular vicious cycle, with allergic muscles causing spasm, spasm causing the build-up of toxic metabolites, and this causing more pain, which the muscles react to with further spasm.

Muscle pain is one of the greatest pains that one can experience. Indeed, labour pains are, of course, muscle pains. Bile stone colic and renal stone colic are also muscle pains – ask any sufferer how bad they are! Muscle pain when accompanied by fatigue is called fibromyalgia. There are several possible explanations, which have implication for treatment:

- Poor energy delivery (through poor mitochondrial, thyroid and adrenal function) results in an early switch into anaerobic metabolism and production of painful lactic acid. This burn may be very prolonged.
- Poor energy delivery also means slow healing and repair.
- Allergic muscles.
- Poor antioxidant status (see page 99).
- Magnesium deficiency – This is necessary for muscles to relax.

Treatment of degenerative-type arthritis and connective tissue problems

- The Basic Package (see page 67)
- Use the tools to treat mechanical problems – structure, friction and wear and tear (see page 110)

Treatment of arthritis where there is inflammation

Examples here include rheumatoid arthritis, sero-negative arthritis, polymyalgia rheumatic and stiff man syndrome.

- As for degenerative-type arthritis (above)
- Try the tools to treat inflammatory conditions and allergy (see page 150)
- Try the tools to treat the upper fermenting gut (see page 102)

Treatment of muscle pain

- All the above
- Tools to tackle energy delivery systems (see page 90)
- Magnesium, possibly by intravenous bolus

V. Pre-conception care and afterwards*

The most important time in life for optimal health and fitness occurs when one is considering starting a family. Nutritional deficiencies, toxic stresses and sub-optimal energy delivery systems, especially hypothyroidism during the three months prior to conception, during pregnancy and breast-feeding, will impact on the growing baby mentally and physically for its lifetime. There will never be a better time to observe the Basic Package (see page 67).

We all start life as one cell composed of our mother's egg and father's sperm. This has to divide into at least 300 different cell types, all within the correct 3D space, and then grow to form an independent human being. This process is exquisitely dependent on good nutritional status and exquisitely sensitive to toxic stress. Simple iodine deficiency resulting in hypothyroidism has massive implications for physical and mental health – babies are born 'cretins'. Even a high-normal TSH level in the mother results in low normal IQ in the baby.

Exposing a foetus to a miniscule dose of the drug thalidomide during the early days of pregnancy may result in seal flipper limbs or 'phocomelia'. Interestingly, thalidomide exerted its effects by its anti-vitamin actions – when tested in animal experiments it was only the vitamin-deficient rats that suffered. In the Western world we are all inevitably polluted by pesticides, toxic metals and other such – perhaps by ensuring excellent nutritional status this will help protect us from the unpredictable malign effects of pollutants.

Mothers treated through pregnancy with the oestrogen mimic stilboestrol increased their lifetime risk of breast cancer by 30 per cent. Their daughters increased their risk of clear cell adenocarcinoma of the vagina and cervix 40-fold. Doctors can be dangerous people!

I give these two examples because they are so obvious. The problem is the less obvious and more subtle occurences. We are seeing epidemics of new problems in children, such as dyslexia, dyspraxia and attention-deficit disorders, together

---

* **Fact:** The male redback spider performs an elaborate courtship dance before conception and then assists the female in her cannibalism of his own body by moving backwards into her mouth, thus ensuring that she enjoys a good meal at the same time. Remarkably only about 20 per cent of male redback spiders ever find a mate.

with serious diseases, such as CFS/ME, autism, Asperger's, type I diabetes and cancer. Autism is estimated to affect 1 per cent of the British population.

Professor Barker followed up babies born in Hertfordshire during the 1930s (the Hertfordshire Cohort Study).[18] They were routinely measured at birth. Babies that had been undernourished during antenatal life were small for dates. Small babies are composed of fewer cells (not smaller cells). These babies grew into adults who were more susceptible to disease and died younger. This was because of organ failures, such as diabetes (pancreatic failure), heart disease and kidney failure. Longevity is determined most by a baby's first 1,000 days within and outside the womb.

The world has its way with us long before we're born.

ANNIE MURPHY PAUL, *Origins: How the Nine Months Before Birth Shape the Rest of Our Lives*

Pre-conceptual care should include detoxification regimes for two reasons. Firstly, the foetus is exquisitely sensitive to toxic stress. Secondly, during breast-feeding the mother will dump about one third of her total body-load of POPs into her breast milk. For example, the Inuit Indians bio-concentrate organo-chlorine pesticides which have bio-accumulated in their food chain – these mothers cannot breast-feed their babies because they develop acute poisoning. For the same reason, weight loss during pregnancy should be avoided – any POPs in fat will be mobilised with the potential to poison the unborn baby.

Birth defects, miscarriages and childhood cancer additionally can be traced back to defects in the father's sperm. Fathers need to do the same regimes as mothers. Foresight (see www.foresight-preconception.org.uk/) have been advising families since 1978, with excellent results with respect to treatment of infertility, recurrent miscarriages and pregnancy outcomes. Results can be seen at www.drmyhill.co.uk/wiki/How_successful_is_the _environmental_approach_to_infertility%3F_Foresight_figures.

What to do

- The Basic Package (see page 67).
- Check rubella antibodies in the mother – It is totally illogical for the NHS to wait until 12 weeks before doing this essential check; by 12 weeks any possible damage has happened.
- If symptoms are present, investigate and treat prior to pregnancy using tools of the trade.
- Stop the contraceptive Pill at least six months before conception.

- Sexually transmitted disease – Many STDs are subclinical with no overt symptoms; these must be identified and eradicated.
- Identify and treat any toxic load – Both parents should consider an assessment of toxic load, including toxic metals in urine following DMSA (see page 197) and a fat biopsy for persistent organic pollutants (POPs). Any detox regime must be done prior to pregnancy. No attempt to detox during pregnancy or breast-feeding should be made, otherwise one simply mobilises toxins and dumps them on the baby.
- Tools for energy delivery (see page 90) – Especially check routinely for and correct hypothyroidism. If this is present, the thyroid should be checked during pregnancy every three months because requirements for thyroid hormones may increase by 50 per cent and poor levels in the mother may result in low IQ in the baby.

For further details see:
www.drmyhill.co.uk/wiki/How_to_ensure_a_healthy_baby

Pregnancy

> Being pregnant is an occupational hazard of being a wife.
>
> QUEEN VICTORIA (1819–1901)

Pregnancy is essential for the propagation of the species but is a dangerous state for the mother. There are high circulating levels of sex hormones, which have properties which are essential to the survival of the baby but detrimental to the health of the mother. These properties are:

- **Blood sugar increase** – To ensure the baby never runs short of energy during critical stages of growth, but this puts the mother at risk of diabetes and metabolic syndrome.
- **Growth promotion** – To ensure rapid growth of the baby – but this will drive an established cancer in the mother.
- **Immune suppression** – This is to prevent rejection of the baby by the maternal immune system, but that puts the mother at increased risk of infection.
- **To induce hypertrophy of smooth muscle in blood vessels and a pro-thrombotic state** – This is to prevent haemorrhage at the time of birth, but puts the mother at risk of eclampsia, deep vein thrombosis (DVT)and pulmonary embolism.

- **Mood destabilisation** – This is to make sure the mother loves the baby so much that its survival becomes more important than her own. Female sex hormones induce a state of madness; Shakespeare recognised this: 'Love is blind, and lovers cannot see the pretty follies that themselves commit' (*Merchant of Venice*).

It is vital to put in place the Basic Package throughout pregnancy to minimise the above risks. We know that low-protein, low-fat and high-carb diets are risk factors for eclampsia (excessively high blood pressure) and can be largely mitigated with a Paleo-ketogenic diet. The most effective treatment of established eclampsia is intravenous magnesium.

What to do throughout pregnancy and breast feeding

Continue all of the above, especially the Basic Package. Mothers are often advised by doctors to stop using micronutrient supplements during pregnancy. Many doctors compare drugs with micronutrients, but this displays a fundamental lack of understanding of biochemistry. Drugs work by blocking enzyme systems and so are intrinsically toxic, whereas micronutrients work by facilitating enzyme systems and so normalise biochemistry and protect against toxic stress. Requirements for micronutrients increase during pregnancy. It is vital they are taken in **proportionate and physiological doses**. It used to be that pregnant women were routinely prescribed high doses of iron during pregnancy – but this blocks zinc absorption with the potential to create other problems.

Paediatrics

All the above that applies to adults also applies to children. But the imperative is greater. Babies and children are developing physically, mentally, emotionally and immunologically. Get things right during these early stages and the child will be set up for rude good health and happiness for life. There will never be a more important time to apply the Basic Package.

We are currently seeing epidemics of adult diseases in children because we are not respecting fundamental evolutionary principles. These include increasingly high rates of: behaviour and developmental disorders (autism, Asperger's, OCD, suicide, eating disorders, hyperactivity), brain disorders (dyslexia, depression, anxiety, personality disorder, psychosis), allergy, auto-immunity, increased bone fracture rates, CFS, premature sexual development with early menarche in girls because of oestrogen mimics, cancer and general ill health. I predict that we will see an era of falling life expectancy as metabolic syndrome takes its toll on the younger generation.

Vaccination

Vaccination is designed to switch on the immune system. The idea is to switch it on against particular microbes, and we call this immunity. However, vaccination may switch on autoimmunity, and probably allergy – it is a two-edged sword. In his preface to Andrew Wakefield's book *Callous Disregard* about vaccination and autism, Dr Peter Fletcher, who was the principal Medical Officer with responsibility for the UK Committee of Safety of Medicines and later Senior Principal Medical Officer and Chief Scientific Officer, wrote of autism:

> . . . it may be that two, or just possibly three, different pathological processes are involved, but the root cause has to be a single initiating factor – almost certainly vaccines.

I recommend that all parents purchase a copy of NHS GP Richard Halvorsen's book *The Truth about Vaccines* so that they can make an informed decision.

VI. Twenty-first century syndromes resulting from increasing environmental pollution

Modern environments have resulted in new syndromes. There is Establishment resistance to recognising these new clinical pictures because to do so would inevitably imply that someone or something is responsible. Such an admission would open up the legal floodgates for compensation. It is an established legal principle (the tort of 'duty of care') that in such cases the polluter should pay. The cheapest and most expedient way to deal with these problems for the Establishment, therefore, is to ignore the sufferers and deny the existence of the syndrome. In this way, the Establishment does not pay for its mistakes and the sufferers have to bear both the health and the financial consequences:

> *Emperors don't stick their necks out. They stick out somebody else's.*
> HANS CHRISTIAN ANDERSEN, *The Emperor's New Clothes*
> (1805–1875)

The twenty-first-century syndromes that I have seen include those listed below. There will be others, arising from the same mechanisms of toxic exposure, immune adjuvants or physical factors I have described, as well perhaps as new types of mechanism as yet unforeseen. But it is a certainty that these syndromes will multiply in number unless we take a stand and refuse to repeat the mistakes of the past:

> The Emperor: 'We'll have your wedding dress made out of the same material.'
> Princess Gilda: 'No!'

HANS CHRISTIAN ANDERSEN (1805–1875)

a. Syndromes switched on by toxic exposures

- **Mercury poisoning** – From exposure to dental amalgam. Mercury is the most toxic element after radioactive elements. It leaks out of fillings from the day they are inserted, with the potential to bio-accumulate in the body.
- **Sick building syndrome** – This is the term for pollution from indoor chemicals: formaldehyde cavity wall insulation, fumes from new carpets, paint, soft furnishings, solvents, plastics, printer fluids, etc. These exposures are often compounded by poor ventilation or recycled air.
- **Gulf War syndrome** – This is triggered by exposure to organophosphate pesticides, oil well fires and biological agents. All these toxicities were worsened by multiple vaccinations.
- **Sheep dip 'flu** – This is triggered by exposure to organo-phosphates and other toxic substances additionally present in sheep dip.
- **Aerotoxic syndrome** – This is seen particularly in pilots and cabin crew and is triggered by exposure to exhaust fumes from jet engines containing noxious gases, burnt volatile organic compounds and organophosphate oil improvers, such as tricreosyl phosphate.
- **9/11 syndrome** – This is seen in fire fighters and is triggered by exposure to burnt plastics (organochlorines) and fire retardants like poly-brominated biphenyls.
  - Carbon monoxide poisoning
  - Fluoride toxicity
  - Pesticide spray drift and garden chemicals
  - House fumigations for fleas
  - Many other possibilities

Being chemically poisoned is like throwing a handful of sand into a finely tuned engine. It wears out faster and has other unexpected effects. Many of these chemicals are persistent and accumulate in fat. Indeed, when I do fat biopsies, results come back in milligrams per kilogram as opposed to blood levels where results are in micrograms per kilogram. This is not a trace level but rather a substantial and clinically significant load.

b. Syndromes switched on by immune adjuvants

- **Silicone implant syndrome** – Silicones leak out from implants from the day they are inserted. They are engulfed by white cells which move throughout the body. These white cells try to digest these tough molecules but are unable to – indeed, there is no biological enzyme that can break down plastic; even my compost heap cannot do such! With luck the immune system chooses to ignore these tough molecules and the potential for harm is low. But for some sensitive women silicone acts as an immune adjuvant to switch on inflammation (burning pain is a feature of siliconosis), allergy and autoimmunity.

c. Syndromes caused by physical factors

- **Wind turbine syndrome** – This has the potential to cause ill health for three reasons:
    Simple noise pollution – a recognised cause of distress, particularly disturbed sleep.
    Amplitude modulation – a palpable wave generated by the blade passing the turbine tower to create a whooshing and disturbing pressure wave.
    Infrasound – This is another wave at very low frequency. It has the potential to resonate with body cavities, setting up standing waves of vibration within. It is not difficult to see how this could greatly disturb internal biochemistry. Many symptoms can be created by infrasound, from fear, sorrow, depression, anxiety, nausea, chest pressure and hallucination to ghostly experiences. Dr Nina Pierpont describes in her book *Wind Turbine Syndrome* vestibular, visceral, vibratory syndrome – this is not memorable except by using a new adjective – patients feel vucking awful!

Clinical features of twenty-first-century syndromes

The clinical picture results from the following mechanisms:

- Acceleration of the metabolic syndrome and the ageing process

- Blockage of energy delivery systems – results in symptoms of CFS/ME
- Switching on inflammation – increased risk of allergy, in particular to chemicals so that multiple chemical sensitivity develops
- Switching on autoimmunity
- Genetic damage – with increased risk of cancer and prion disorders; offspring of poisoned parents are at greater risk of abnormalities
- Growth-promoting effects – ability to promote cancer and prion disorders

Treatment

It is essential to recognise and address the underlying cause. Doing this over my clinical career has turned me into an environmental campaigner and landed me into terrible trouble with the received Establishment thinking. The problem is that patients suffering from these severe diseases do not have the resources of energy, money or time to fight. It is a fact that the Establishment abides by Roger Stone's 'Three Corollaries': 'Admit nothing, deny everything, launch counterattack.'

For my part, I treat the sufferers to the best of my ability and, oh yes, I abide by just the third corollary of Stone's. This book is part of my counterattack.

Other treatment options include:

- Tools to treat metabolic syndrome – Employ the Basic Package (see page 67)
- Tools for detoxification (see page 105) – Even after the cause of the problem has been removed, it is possible to be reacting to chemicals stored in the body
- Tools to address energy delivery systems (see page 90)
- Tools to treat inflammatory conditions (see page 89) – notably allergy and autoimmunity

The above list will never be comprehensive as new syndromes come to light. This is not important, in itself, so long as the underlying mechanisms are identified and the relevant tools are put in place.

The next chapter follows with case histories which illustrate the power of ecological medicine to treat serious disease using logical and fundamentally safe interventions.

CHAPTER 5

Case histories

I. Living to one's full potential: Jeanne Calment (21 February 1875 – 4 August 1997)

Jeanne Louise Calment was a French woman who had the longest confirmed human lifespan in history, by living to the age of 122. She had good health throughout life by dint of an excellent diet, exercise and lifestyle. At age 85, she took up fencing and rode her bicycle up until her 100th birthday. Calment lived on her own until shortly before her 110th birthday, when she needed to be moved to a nursing home following a cooking accident when, through problems with sight, she started a small fire in her house. However, she remained in good shape, and continued to walk until she fractured her femur in a fall at the age of 114 years, which required surgery.

Calment did everything in moderation – she smoked from the age of 21 (1896) to 117 (1992), but just two cigarettes per day. She was slim, weighing just 45 kilograms (99 lb) in 1994. She ascribed her longevity and relatively youthful appearance for her age to olive oil, which she said she poured on all her food and rubbed onto her skin, as well as enjoying port wine and chocolate. Every year on her birthday she regaled reporters with quips about her secret of longevity – the list changed each year and included laughter, activity and 'a stomach like an ostrich's'. She obviously did not suffer from fermenting gut!

She was said to be – constitutionally and biologically speaking – immune to stress: 'If you can't do anything about it, don't worry about it.' However, she did not have a stressful life – her husband was wealthy and this made it possible for Calment never to have to work; instead she led a leisured lifestyle, pursuing hobbies such as tennis, cycling, swimming, roller-skating, piano and opera. She aged well: 'I've never had but one wrinkle, and I'm sitting on it'.

Clearly Calment did not have metabolic syndrome; she powered her body with fat (olive oil and high-fat chocolate), not carbohydrates; she did not need addictions to cope with stress, neither did she suffer diseases associated with inflammation. Her mother lived to 86 and so she had inherited her good mitochondria. Perhaps most importantly, apart from her fracture, she managed to avoid doctors and hospitals.

II. A case of cancer:
Carwen and chronic lymphatic leukaemia (CLL)

Carwen came to my surgery in January 2004, then aged 69, with a droopy left eyelid – a nerve palsy called Horner's syndrome. This was confirmed by a consultant neurologist. Routine blood tests then demonstrated she also had chronic lymphatic leukaemia with a high lymphocyte (white blood cell) count of $11.04 \times 109/1$ (1.5–4.0); this diagnosis was confirmed by a consultant haematologist, but the white cell count was not sufficiently high to merit chemotherapy. She was prescribed steroids for her Horner's syndrome, which thankfully resolved it, and her lymphocyte count dropped to $6.49 \times 109/1$. She was also noted to have a right-sided cataract. Blood tests also showed borderline hypothyroidism with a free T4 of 8.6 pmol/l (12–22), so I started her on thyroxin.

With any tumour I like to have a tumour marker so that one can assess progress. In CLL the lymphocyte count is such a marker. This meant we were able closely to monitor Carwen's response to nutritional and detoxification therapies.

She started the Basic Package of treatment (Paleo-ketogenic diet, nutritional supplements, exercise – see page 67), combined with monthly vitamin B12 injections. Cancer cells can only live on sugar, and so a low-GI (glycaemic index – see page 130) diet was critical. Dairy products contain natural growth promoters and so these too were cut out. It was not, and is still not, easy. Carwen was a keen member of the local Women's Institute and every function was accompanied by breads, cakes, biscuits, pastas, pies and quiches, all of which were forbidden foods.

Despite sticking to the diet, and gradually losing weight, the lymphocyte count continued to creep up.

In September 2005 we tested for DNA adducts (see page 198). This is a test of substances 'stuck onto DNA'. Of course, nothing should be 'stuck on' – DNA should be pristine. We found the presence of the insecticide lindane 'stuck onto' Carwen's DNA at a level of 17 ng/ml. This was a breakthrough. Lindane is a known carcinogen and a problem for at least two reasons. Firstly, it may block genes or up-regulate them. Carcinogenesis could result from the blocking of genes that control growth, or those that control the synthesis of proteins responsible for DNA repair, or other mechanisms. Secondly, lindane has oestrogenic-like properties – and oestrogen is a growth promoter.

Where there is a problem like this with a chemical we have to ask both where the chemical came from and also how it can be removed from the body. In Carwen's case, lindane probably came from an episode in 1977 when she treated inherited furniture for woodworm. Since then lindane has been banned as a timber treatment because it is so toxic.

I have done some sort of test of toxicity on 27 patients, before and after sauna sweating regimes, and I know that levels of pesticide and volatile organic compounds (VOCs) come down reliably well with this regime. Because Carwen was not a CFS patient (we treat them with far-infrared sauna-ing – see page 82) and we had a local facility, Carwen started traditional sauna-ing techniques on a twice-weekly basis.

In March 2006 we repeated the DNA adducts test and there was still 11 ng/ml of lindane present. Carwen increased her sauna-ing to three times a week and in September 2006 DNA adducts showed just a trace of lindane present. This was commented on by the lab as 'excellent progress'. The enzyme responsible for healing DNA is zinc-dependent. In the original biopsy, zinc levels were just 27 ng/ml (normal range 21–74 ng/ml), but this had now come up nicely to 44 ng/ml.

During the course of the above regimes, Carwen progressively lost weight from 15 stone 7 lb to 12 stone 5 lb. During this time we plotted lymphocyte counts and graphed them and that graph is given below. The normal range for lymphocytes (1.0–4.0 × 109/l) lies below this scale.

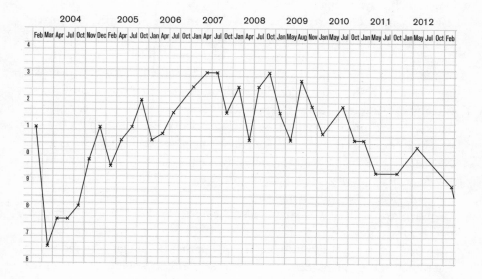

The lymphocyte count increased progressively from 2004, reaching a peak in 2007. During this time Carwen had lindane on her DNA which could have acted as a growth promoter. Furthermore, she really struggled to do the diet and it was not fully established until 2007. Her lymphocyte count stayed fairly constant until 2009, since when it has fallen progressively. This fall was initially achieved with no conventional therapy, simply Paleo-ketogenic diet, including avoiding dairy products and carbohydrates, plus vitamin B12 injections, increasing exercise and of course the detox sauna-ing. In summary, the tools of the trade that we used were:

The Basic Package (see page 67)
Tools to detoxify (see page 106)
Tools to treat abnormal growths (see page 113)

Although the diet was hard work, Carwen felt very much better in herself. Her energy levels were improved, a problem she had with falling asleep at functions disappeared (narcolepsy is commonly caused by intolerance of gluten grains), chronic catarrh disappeared (probably dairy allergy) and an intolerance of sunlight improved so she no longer needed to wear dark glasses. A recent trip to the optician showed that her cataract had not become any worse. Interestingly, her optician reported that her visual acuity had improved by 3 dioptres and commented that it was most unusual for visual acuity to get better.

However, during this time Carwen continued to suffer the odd flare of a long-standing eye problem – iritis – with a flare in May 2012. The iritis had started following the birth of her only child and she had suffered recurrent attacks since. With every attack of iritis her lymphocyte count spiked, which I thought was probably a viral response, so partly because of this and partly out of scientific curiosity, I decided to start her on the anti-viral drug acyclovir (800 mg five times daily) and referred her back to her consultant ophthalmologist. What was so interesting was that not only did her iritis clear up very quickly, but she felt so much better again, over and above previous improvements. When we repeated the lymphocyte count it had dropped to as low as it had ever been – to $8.7 \times 10^9/l$. More recently it fell again to $7.4 \times 10^9/l$. On the advice of her consultant ophthalmologist, we decided to continue with long-term low-dose acyclovir 400 mg daily.

At her last visit to the haematologist, the doctor said to Carwen, 'I am puzzled as to why you are so well.'

I suspect that Carwen picked up a virus during her pregnancy and that it had caused her problems for years, initially with iritis, possibly as a cause of her

Horner's syndrome, and more recently as one factor in driving her CLL. This illustrates the point that pregnancy may result in mild immunosuppression, with a chance for viruses to become established. It may well be that chronic lymphatic leukaemia has a viral element and that taking anti-virals over and above the other interventions has been additionally helpful.

It is also worth noting that Carwen reports continuing to feel extremely well in herself, indeed much fitter than most of her peers, who are disbelieving when she informs them that she is suffering from leukaemia. Carwen is a singer – with acyclovir she has also found her singing voice much improved as previously she had lost clarity and pitch.

However, I know the battle is not over – it is a war, well fought, that Carwen is winning. She is now 78. She feels as fit as she has ever been and is intellectually sharp. Most importantly, she is highly motivated and, with a bit of kicking from me (metaphorical rather than actual I hasten to add!), sticking to the regimes. I see no reason why she should not continue to do well.

III. A case of Gulf War syndrome: Joseph

Joe was referred to me in 2005 for treatment of his Gulf War syndrome. The two so-called 'Gulf Wars' were the most toxic wars in history. All the pro-inflammatory infectious and toxic problems of modern Western lives were compressed into a few months. Young men, who were not allowed to become soldiers unless they were 100 per cent fit and well, were rendered sick for life. Joe tells me that he and others were subject to a combination of extensive vaccination, toxic chemicals (including pesticides like organophosphates and pyrethroids; also dioxins, flame retardants, tributyl tin and so on), chemicals from burning oil-well fires, contaminated drinking water, radiation exposures from depleted uranium used in warheads, and probably stealth biological warfare – notably *Mycoplasma incognito*.

All the above factors would be expected to accelerate the rate of degeneration and switch on autoimmunity, allergy and cancer.

Joe presented with a clinical picture of chronic fatigue syndrome, chronic obstructive airway's disease, rosacea, scleroderma (his forearm felt solid, like a lump of wood) and multiple allergies to chemicals and foods.

Where there is such a complex clinical picture, it is almost impossible to tease out the different threads of mechanisms. Indeed, when one mechanism goes down so do others. So in this case we simply had to put in place as much of the package of treatment as possible. In this respect, Joe has been incredibly well motivated and disciplined and without that discipline I doubt he would be alive today.

A fat biopsy in 2005 showed the presence of organophosphates, tributyl tin, PCBs, lindane and DDD. DNA adducts showed high levels of benzene and tin with very low levels of zinc. So we put in place the tools of the trade as follows:

The Basic Package (see page 67)
Tools to improve energy delivery (see page 90) – coenzyme Q10,
    D-ribose, acetyl-L-carnitine, vitamin B3, magnesium and B12
    injections, to support mitchondria
Tools to detoxify (see page 106) – including far-infrared (FIR) sauna-ing
Tools to damp down inflammation and put out the biochemical fire
    (see page 66) – including enzyme potentiated desensitisation (EPD)

Joe was markedly intolerant of the compound I use for toxic metal chelation – DMSA – so we had to rely on nutritional supplements, including glutathione, to reduce the toxic metals.

In 2006, before the benefits of the above could be fully realised, Joe developed malignant hypertension with encephalopathy and renal failure. He spent 14 days in intensive care and was unconscious for 5 days. He was treated with high-dose steroids, antibiotics, anti-hypertensives, warfarin and anti-epileptic drugs. It was extraordinary that he survived – he should have died.

On discharge he was taking a shopping list of medication. He was on the waiting list for renal dialysis with a glomerular filtration rate of 19 ml/min. This is late-stage renal failure.

Once home, Joe was able to put back in place his regime of diet, nutritional supplements and detoxification. Since then he has gradually improved. His scleroderma improved to the extent that the skin of his forearms became soft again. His blood pressure normalised and so we were able to stop much of his medication. This improvement has been paralleled by improving renal function, as charted by his creatinine levels on page 177.

There have been additional tools put in place as I have learned more – namely:

Tools for the fermenting gut: Joe suffered very much from abdominal bloating despite doing an excellent Paleo-ketogenic diet. We decided to cut out all carbohydrates ruthlessly – he had to swap from powering his body with carbs to powering it with fat. This had some interesting effects. Joe lost 10lb of weight in less than a week; I suspect much of this was allergic oedema. His bloating ceased as did the noisy rumbling gut. His rosacea improved markedly.

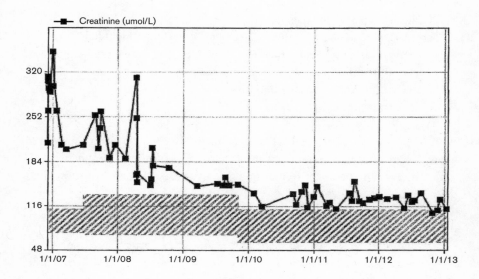

Intravenous magnesium bolus injections – These, delivered at his home, greatly improved energy and well-being. They also improved his lung function.

Joe is not currently taking any regular prescription medication; he just takes nutritional supplements. He does need antibiotics and steroids to control his asthma flares. He still has to pace his activities in order to feel well. He is highly disciplined with his diet, nutritional supplements, avoidance of chemicals and detox regimes, but life is very much worth living again!

IV. A case of multiple allergies, heart disease and cancer: Patricia

Patricia was referred to me by Dr John Mansfield in 2003 following his retirement. He had much improved her arthritis with desensitising neutralisation injections. We continued desensitisation with enzyme potentiated desensitisation (EPD) and she did well.

Patricia had been diagnosed with heart block in 1993, requiring a pacemaker. Interestingly, this had followed a viral infection. She was then aged 71.

In 2005, aged 83, Patricia developed breast cancer. She was deemed not fit for surgery and treated with chemotherapy. However, this made her acutely ill, she developed heart failure and chemotherapy had to be halted. This was the stimulus to put in place the major tools of the trade:

The Basic Package (see page 67).

Tools to improve energy delivery (see page 90) – These included intravenous magnesium injections, which proved to be very helpful.

Tools to treat inflammatory conditions (see page 66) – Love and laughter proved especially helpful!

Tools to treat abnormal growths.

Patricia developed an irritable bladder which disturbed her sleep. I suspected allergy to gut flora and so we put in place the tools to improve gut function with emphasis on the upper fermenting gut. Even today this includes low-dose daily antibiotics.

Patricia continued to be monitored at the breast clinic. Her breast cancer did not grow or spread. However, it was decided to try an aromatase inhibitor – arimidex. This worsened her heart failure and so this drug was stopped.

It was clear that autumn was a bad time for Patricia; she always relapsed at this time of year. This is typical of mould allergy. So mould filters were purchased for her living room and bedroom and this improved matters further. Indeed, I referred her to Dr David Freed for neutralisation for moulds, and thankfully this was helpful and much improved her low mood.

Things ticked over reasonably well until March 2011 when she fell and broke her hip. She was denied surgery and for six months lived with a broken hip. This was a terrible and painful time, but she refused to die. She lived on morphine. During this time her breast cancer grew, but did not spread. Eventually, she persuaded a surgeon to operate, promising not to sue him if she died! Her hip was pinned and plated, twice, so she was again able to travel to me for her magnesium injections. She was able to stop her morphine and her breast cancer shrank.

Patricia continued to see me regularly for magnesium and B12 injections until very sadly she fell and fractured her hip, and died at the age of 93. She was witty and funny right to the very end. If I slipped up on a point of fact, I was immediately put right.

V. A case of inflammatory arthritis: Jo and polymyalgia rheumatica

Jo is a friend and fellow team chaser (horse racing in teams over cross-country fences). She had been fit and well until 2005 when, aged 57, she developed polymyalgia rheumatic (PMR) – a nasty inflammatory arthropathy. She had a raised erythrocyte sedimentation rate (ESR) of 34 mm/hour which rose to

97 mm/hour. She was prescribed high-dose steroids, but these made her feel muzzy headed and spaced out. She was unable to ride and was reduced to hobbling around.

Jo undertook the Basic Package of Paleo-ketogenic diet and nutritional supplements. She was also diagnosed with borderline osteoporosis and therefore judiciously took high-dose vitamin D and strontium 250 mg daily. As a result of these interventions, her ESR came down to 30 mm/hour, but she was still experiencing constant muscle aching.

At this stage I suspected allergy to gut microbes and so she did a comprehensive digestive stool analysis. This showed the presence of six additional species of bacteria that I would not expect to find, all at high levels. Therefore she started on a zero-starch diet. After her third week on a starch-free diet, Jo sent me an email: 'The result is nothing short of miraculous. The muscle pain is very much better!' Three months later Jo's PMR aches returned and her ESR spiked up to 48 mm/hour. She confessed that she had lapsed on the low-starch diet because new potato, carrot and beetroot had become available. Again she toughened up on the diet, back onto her low-starch regime, and her muscle aches disappeared. By the autumn of 2012 she was able to ride and start competing in our sport of team chasing.

Her bone density scans results are as follows:

21/01/2011	28/03/2013
Lumbar spine 0.895	Lumbar spine 0.950
Femoral neck 0.751	Femoral neck 0.779

Doctors expect bone density to decline with age. The regimes I recommended have increased Jo's bone density simply by taking nutritional supplements.

Jo has now taken on Mastership of the Atherstone Hunt, which means at least twice-weekly long days in the saddle following and keeping up with a Huntsman, who is less than half her age.

In conclusion, Jo was treated with:

The Basic Package (see page 67)
Tools to treat inflammation (see page 66)
Tools to treat mechanical problems (see page 110)
Tools for improving gut function (see page 201), especially the
     fermenting gut

VI. A case of CFS: Peter

CFS is one of the worst-treated conditions – it is the classic example of what happens when patients, often encouraged by their doctors, ignore symptoms. Fatigue is the symptom that protects us from ourselves, and when we experience it we often mask it with addiction (caffeine, alcohol, pain killers, etc). We then carry on with sheer bloody-mindedness and so the people who go on to develop CFS are often the workaholic, perfectionist, goal-driven characters. This personality that gets one into CFS does not allow one to escape.

We cannot solve our problems with the same thinking we used when we created them.

ALBERT EINSTEIN (1879–1955)

Whilst there are obvious triggers to CFS, such as viral infection or chemical exposure, almost always there is a build-up period of high-intensity, unremitting stress. Peter was a classic example of this. He worked in a high-powered job as an accountant, dealing with international issues. He found that from 2001 he really had to push himself mentally and physically to function to his full potential. In October 2002, he picked up an ear infection which resulted in a complete physical breakdown; he could not function for months. He made a slight recovery, then got glandular fever, relapsed and reached a very low plateau which he described as being 'in hibernation'. This persisted for years until he came to see me in March 2007.

The tools we used were:

The Basic Package (see page 67)
Tools to treat poor energy delivery (see page 90)

Peter had a very poor mitochondrial energy score of 0.10, which means he had just 10 per cent of the energy available to cells compared to the lowest limit of the normal range. These tests were characterised by severe blocking of translocator protein function and ADP to ATP conversion – indeed, even now the latter figure was a record high. Translocator function tests showed blocking by dichlorobenzene, DNA/RNA (probably viral) and glutathione conjugates. Therefore, in addition to supplements to correct mitochondrial function we put in place:

Tools to detoxify (see page 106) – particularly FIR sauna (see page 82)

Peter had low-normal levels of free T4, indicating underactive thyroid, and so thyroxin was added into the regime.

By October 2007, the mitochondrial function tests had improved, with an energy score of 0.54 (and subsequently in November 2011 the score was better again: 0.70). However, the biochemical improvement was not paralleled by clinical improvements. We had to look elsewhere for the causes of his CFS.

Upper fermenting gut is very common in CFS. A urine test showed the presence of hydrogen sulphide, suggesting fermentation by bacteria, and also high levels of arabinose, typical of yeast fermentation. There were also high levels of short-chain polypeptides in the blood, suggesting leaky gut. So we put in place:

Tools to improve gut function (see page 102) – particularly anti-fungals to treat fermenting gut by yeast.

Peter stuck to the difficult regimes to the letter and with great determination, but he was just not getting the clinical result I expected. This was starting to give me sleepless nights too! We then had a bit of a clue – unsure whether the thyroxin was helping we tried stopping it. Peter seemed to get a little worse. About this time I was learning about thyroid hormone receptor resistance and so we decided that a trial of pure T3 was in order. This was started in February 2012.

Since then there has been progressive improvement. Peter coped with the freezing winter of 2012/13 better than expected, started to play indoor tennis (two sets maximum), managed a skiing holiday and a trip to France. Crashes of energy were increasingly rare and brief in duration. This was a huge improvement clinically. He reckons he is now functioning at 75–80 per cent of his potential.

This history illustrates the importance of the combined nutritional/hormonal/detox approach. Thyroid hormones manifest through their effects on mitochondria – had we not corrected the mitochondrial problem first there would have been no response to pure T3. Furthermore, despite not identifying the viral DNA/RNA stuck onto translocator protein (and I still do not know what to do about such a finding), Peter was still able to recover. Give the immune system the raw materials and energy and it can cope with much.

VII. A case of infertility: Agnes

Agnes came to see me in December 2008, aged 42, wishing to start a family. She had previously conceived but had been unable to sustain a pregnancy. She knew much about the importance of diet and good nutrition and so much of the Basic Package was already in place. However, the elephant in the room became apparent from her history – she worked as a restorer of stained-glass windows and so she was occupationally exposed to toxic metals which were used to stain the glass. Blood tests also showed that she was hypothyroid and so thyroxin was started. A measure of fertility, anti-mullerian hormone, was low, suggesting her fertility was low, so I was not too hopeful of success.

DNA adducts in December 2008 showed the presence of three toxic metals present on her DNA – namely lead, nickel and cobalt. These were at high levels. So we put in place the tools to detoxify. Because time was at a premium, Agnes did it all – sauna-ing and oral chelation therapy with DMSA, together with the nutritional supplements and normalising thyroid function. Repeat DNA adducts in April 2009 showed no lead or cobalt, but some nickel remained. Agnes carried on detoxing.

Agnes's partner, Jim, joined in with the detox techniques and his sperm count improved markedly between July 2008 and June 2010, with the count rising from 29 million / ml to 75 million / ml, with all other parameters also improving.

Agnes and Jim decided not to use any artificial methods of conceiving but trust to Mother Nature. In January 2012 Agnes delivered a healthy boy, Ben, weighing 8 lb 4 oz. Agnes was 46 and very happy!

Postscript

Western Medicine has lost its way. Doctors no longer look for the underlying causes of disease, a process which used to be called diagnosis, but rather seek a 'quick fix' response that will see the patient out of their surgery door in under 10 minutes. This quick fix response usually comprises the prescribing of symptom suppressing medications. Doctors have become the puppets of Big Pharma, dishing out drugs and working to a 'checklist' culture which is directed at the symptom rather than the patient. Patients are seen as a collection of walking symptoms, rather than as people, each with a highly individual set of circumstances. Worse than this, not only do these prescription drugs do nothing to address the root causes of illness, but often they accelerate the underlying pathology and so drug prescribing snowballs. This leads to a vicious spiral of increasing drug costs, coupled with worsening pathologies for individual patients, whilst at the same time there is an increasing number of new, and chronic, patients because their illnesses are never properly addressed at the root cause. It is no wonder that the National Health Service is being overwhelmed. The result is that millions suffer a painful, premature, and often lingering, death from diseases which are completely avoidable and reversible.

The time has come for patients to be empowered, by taking back control of their own health. To achieve this empowerment, patients need:

1. The knowledge to work out why they have symptoms and disease.
2. Direct access to all relevant medical tests.
3. Direct access to knowledgeable health practitioners who can further advise and guide them, together with direct access to safe and effective remedies.

None of this is beyond patients who are always highly motivated to be well again, and who always know their bodies better than anyone else. It is time to break down the artificial barriers that have been placed between patients and the direct access to medical knowledge, tests and experts that they so deserve. This three-stage process of patient emancipation is addressed in the following ways:

1. The knowledge can be found in my four books:
    a) *Sustainable Medicine: whistle-blowing on 21st century medical practices.* This book – which I hope you are either about to read or are reading now – is the starting point for treating all symptoms and diseases. It explains why we have symptoms, such as fatigue and pain, and explains how we can work out the mechanisms of such symptoms and which are the appropriate medical tests to diagnose these mechanisms. Most importantly, *Sustainable Medicine* identifies the 'Tools of the Trade' to effect a cure. These tools include diet, nutritional supplements and natural remedies.
    b) *Prevent and Cure Diabetes: delicious diets, not dangerous drugs.* All medical therapies should start with diet. Modern Western diets are driving our modern epidemics of diabetes, heart disease, cancer and dementia – this process is called metabolic syndrome. *Prevent and Cure Diabetes* explains in detail why and how we have arrived at a situation where the real weapons of mass destruction can be found in our own kitchens. Importantly, it describes the vital steps every one of us can make to reverse this situation so that life can be lived to its full potential.
    c) *Diagnosis and Treatment of Chronic Fatigue Syndrome and Myalgic Encephalitis: it's mitochondria, not hypochondria: Second Edition.* This book further explores the commonest symptom which people complain of, namely fatigue, together with its pathological end result when this symptom is ignored. This is my life's work, having spent over 35 years in clinical practice, many months doing academic research and co-authored three scientific papers, all directed at solving this jigsaw of an illness. This book has application not just for the severely fatigued patient but also for the athlete looking for peak performance and for anybody not feeling on top form.
    d) *The PK Cookbook: go Paleo-ketogenic and get the best of both worlds.* This gives us the *how* of the PK (Paleo-ketogenic) diet. This is the starting point for preventing and treating modern Western diseases, including diabetes, arterial disease, dementia and cancer. Dietary changes are always the most difficult, but also the most important, intervention. This book is based on my first-hand experience and research on developing a PK diet that is sustainable long term. Perhaps the most

important feature of this diet is the PK bread – this has helped more
people stick to this diet than all else! Secondly, the book introduces
PK salt (named Sunshine salt because it is rich in vitamin D). This
salt is comprised of all essential minerals (plus vitamins D and B12)
in physiological amounts within a sea salt. This more than compensates for the mineral deficiencies that are ubiquitously present
in all foods from Western agricultural systems. It is an essential and
delicious addition to all modern Western diets.

2. Access to medical tests
   Many medical tests can be accessed directly through www.blood
       testsdirect.co.uk
   Here blood tests can be accessed directly without a doctor's request.
       Many can be done on finger-drop samples of blood. www.armin
       labs.com/en
   These blood tests (including for Lyme disease) can be accessed
       directly without the need for a referral from a doctor or other
       health practitioner. www.biolab.co.uk
   For these tests you need referral by a health practitioner – see
       'NHW' below. www.gdx.net/uk
   This is the link for Genova labs – referral by a health practitioner is
       needed - see 'NHW' below.
   Tests include blood, urine, stool and saliva samples. Many blood tests
   can be carried out at home on a finger-drop sample of blood, without
   the need for a nurse or doctor to be involved at all.

3. Direct access to knowledgeable health practitioners who can further
   advise and guide patients
   Natural Health Worldwide (NHW) is a website where any knowl-
       edgeable practitioner (experienced patient, health professional
       or doctor) can offer their opinion to any patient. This opinion
       may be free, or for a fee, by telephone, email, or Skype. The
       Practitioner needs no premises or support staff since bookings
       and payments are made online. Patients give feedback to that
       Practitioner's Reputation page and star ratings evolve. See www
       .naturalhealthworldwide.com

Recommended reading

Baillie-Hamilton P. *The Detox Diet: eliminate chemical calories and restore your body's natural slimming system*. London, UK: Michael Joseph; 2002.

Dawkins R. *The Selfish Gene* 2nd ed. Oxford, UK: Oxford Paperbacks; 1989.

Dawkins R. *The Extended Phenotype: the long reach of the gene*. Oxford, UK: Oxford Paperbacks; 1999.

Gotzsche PC. *Mammography Screening: truth, lies and controversy*. London: Radcliffe Publishing Ltd; 2012.

Groves B. *Trick and Treat: how 'healthy eating' is making us ill*. London: Hammersmith Press; 2010.

Halvorsen R. *The Truth about Vaccines: making the right decision for your child*. London: Gibson Square Books; 2009.

Kaufman W. *The Common Cause of Joint Dysfunction*. 1949.

Lane N. *Power, Sex, Suicide: mitochondria and the meaning of life*. Oxford, UK: OUP; 2006.

Little JR, McGuff D. *Body by Science: a research-based program for strength training, body building, and complete fitness in 12 minutes a week*. New York: McGraw-Hill; 2009.

Myhill S. *Diagnosis and Treatment of Chronic Fatigue Syndrome: it's mitochondria, not hypochondria*. White River Junction, VT: Chelsea Green Publishing; 2018.

Plant J. *Your Life in Your Hands: understand, prevent and overcome breast cancer and ovarian cancer*. London: Virgin Books; 2007.

Robinson P. *Recovering with T3: my journey from hypothyroidism to good health using the T3 thyroid hormone*. Elephant in the Room Books; 2013.

Rogers SA. *Detoxify or Die*. Sarasota, FL: Sand Key Company; 2002.

Sinatra S. *The Sinatra Solution: metabolic cardiology*. Laguna Beach, CA: Basic Health Publications; 2011.

Stalmatski A. *Freedom from Asthma: Buteyko's revolutionary treatment*. London: Kyle Cathie; 1999.

Walker M. 'The Persecution and Resistance of Loïc le Ribault'. *Nexus Magazine* volume 12; issues 3 and 4. www.whale.to/b/walker2.html.

Glossary

Acid–alkali balance

Maintaining the correct acidity/alkalinity (or pH) of the blood is an essential part of good health. Acidity/alkalinity is determined by the concentration of hydrogen ions – that is, the lower the pH, the greater the acidity and the greater the concentration of hydrogen ions. It is important to realise the pH scale is a logarithmic one. This means that the difference between a pH of 7 and 4 is a thousand-fold increase in hydrogen ions. (For the mathematically minded, this is calculated, in this case, as $7 - 4 = 3$, and then raising 10 to the power of 3, giving 1000.) Such a shift would have a massive effect on biochemical processes, most of which are exquisitely sensitive to pH changes. For normal metabolism, the pH of the blood is tightly controlled by the lungs and the kidneys. In the short term, the lungs compensate where there is a tendency to acidosis (increased acidity) by slowing breathing and thereby retaining carbon dioxide and increasing bicarbonate, and with that, the pH. In the medium term, the kidneys compensate – where there is acidosis, we pee out acid.

This works fine when we have enough acid or bicarbonate to play with. We run into problems when we don't. Where there is poor mitochondrial function, we slip into anaerobic metabolism and produce lactic acid. This chronic overproduction puts us into a permanently acidic state, which means that any person with a tendency to fatigue and anaerobic metabolism is likely to be chronically acidotic. We try to correct this by peeing out acid, but there is only so much we can do.

I suspect the upper fermenting gut results in an acidosis – sugars may be fermented into acids, such as D-lactate, to cause D-lactate acidosis.

The possible effects of being acidic are:

- Hypoglycaemia – An acidic body means we cannot release glucose from the liver, nor can we make use of sugar in blood and muscle (glycolysis, that is the conversion of glucose, is inhibited). So mitochondria are further starved of energy and the sufferer craves carbs, feeling ghastly when he/she does not eat.
- Muscles contract less strongly.

- Acid urine strips out minerals so we lose minerals too easily. Acidic urine is a risk factor for osteoporosis.
- Plasma potassium levels may rise.

Hyperventilation will worsen any tendency to acidosis because it washes out carbon dioxide, and therefore bicarbonate, from the blood.

http://www.drmyhill.co.uk/wiki/Acid-Alkali_balance

Acquired metabolic dyslexias

As we age, just like an ageing car, we become less efficient in three respects. Firstly, we need more raw materials as our ability to digest and absorb declines. Those that I currently believe need to be supplemented in supra-physiological doses include vitamin B12 1 mg, vitamin B3 500 mg, vitamin D 2,000 IU and vitamin C 2 g. There may well be others. Secondly, our ability to synthesise key molecules from raw materials declines. My list of such so far includes melatonin (the sleep hormone – 3 mg), adrenal hormones (such as pregnenolone – 50 mg, possibly, and DHEA), coenzyme Q10 (200 mg) and D-ribose (5 g). Again, there may well be others as I learn more. Thirdly, we need additional help with detoxification since we live in an increasingly toxic world. I consider glutathione (250 mg daily) to be essential.

ADP and ATP (adenosine diphosphate and adenosine triphosphate)

ATP is the energy molecule necessary to power almost everything that happens in the body, from contracting a muscle to synthesising a hormone and generating a nerve signal. In releasing its energy, it is converted to ADP. ADP is recycled back to ATP by the engines of our cells called mitochondria through a process called oxidative phosphorylation.

Adrenal gland problems

The adrenal gland is the 'gear box' of our car responsible for matching energy demand with energy consumption. It is additionally responsible for controlling the amount of inflammation in the body. It achieves this by secreting adrenaline (the short-term response, measured in seconds and minutes), followed by cortisol (a medium-term response, measured in minutes and hours), followed by DHEA (dehydroepiandrosterone – a longer-term stress hormone).

The Hungarian physiologist Hans Selye showed that if you stressed rats, their adrenal glands enlarged to produce more stress hormones (including cortisol and DHEA) to allow the rat to cope with that stress. If the rat had a break and a rest, then the adrenal gland would return to its normal size and recover. However, if the rat was stressed without a break or a rest, he would be apparently all right for some time, but then suddenly collapse and die. When Selye looked at the adrenal glands at this point, they were shrivelled up. The glands had become exhausted.

The current Western way of life is for people to push themselves more and more. Many can cope with a great deal of stress, but everybody has their breaking point. The adrenal gland is responsible for the body's hormonal response to this stress. It produces adrenaline, which stimulates the instant stress hormone response ('fight or flight' reaction), and cortisol and DHEA, which create the medium- and long-term stress hormone responses respectively. When the gland becomes exhausted, chronic fatigue develops and tests of adrenal function typically show low levels of cortisol and DHEA. DHEA has only recently been studied because it had not been realised that it had any important actions.

All steroid hormone synthesis starts with cholesterol. The first biochemical step takes place in mitochondria where there is a conversion to pregnenolone. The body can then shunt from pregnenolone into either a stress or catabolic mode (to cortisol) or a rebuilding mode (anabolic hormones such as DHEA, testosterone and oestrogen).

Both anabolism (building up tissues) and catabolism (breaking tissues down) are essential for life in the right amounts: too little causes problems, as does too much. Research suggests this balance protects against the development of osteoporosis, which is a major consideration for anyone unable to exercise, including all CFS sufferers.

http://drmyhill.co.uk/wiki/Common_Hormonal_Problems_in_CFS

Advanced glycation end products

These are the damaged goods produced when sugar sticks to other molecules, which could be proteins or fats or other such. They are a major cause of arterial damage. Increasingly there is evidence suggesting they stick to proteins in the nervous system to form prions and so drive neurological diseases like Alzheimer's and Parkinson's disease.

Aerotoxic syndrome

The poisoning of airline pilots, cabin crew and passengers is possible in any air flight! Over the past few decades there has been a fundamental design fault in the majority of airplanes used to move people around the world. The engines compress and heat outside air which is then mixed with fuel and burned in order to propel the aircraft.

As the air is already compressed and warmed, it makes for a cheap way of supplying breathing air to the cabin. However, it is subject to contamination from the engines particularly if engine design is faulty or if engine seals become worn. Indeed, all engines leak oils and fumes to a certain extent, especially as they age, and these chemicals get in to cabin air. Because jet engines run at such high temperatures, additives are put into oil so they can work better. Therefore depending on the design, the age and the recent service history of the engine, occupants of any aircraft will be more or less poisoned by these fumes.

http://www.drmyhill.co.uk/wiki/Aerotoxic_syndrome
http://www.aerotoxic.org

Allergic muscles

Allergy never ceases to surprise and amaze me for the multiplicity of symptoms that it can cause. It is now clear to me that any part of the body can react allergically. Irritable bowel syndrome is partly due to allergy in the gut, migraine is allergy in the brain, asthma is allergy in the lungs, so why not allergic muscles? The more I look for this condition the more I find it, and it is obvious when you look for it.

The natural progression of allergy is for allergens to start producing symptoms in one target organ and move on to another. So the typical history through life of the dairy allergic person would be to start with colic as a baby, then move on to other manifestations such as toddler diarrhoea, catarrh, ear infections and sore throats, irritable bowel syndrome, migraine, arthritis, fatigue and allergic muscles.

How do allergic muscles start? What seems to happen is that muscles get sensitised as a result of mechanical damage. Tearing or bruising the muscle means that it comes in direct contact with blood, which may be carrying food antigens. I suspect the allergy is switched on at that time and the pain which follows the muscle damage and which persists long term is mis-attributed to damage, when actually it is sensitisation. So a torn muscle in the back from, say, lifting a heavy load could sensitise to, say, dairy products and it is the consumption of dairy subsequently which keeps the problem on the boil.

http://drmyhill.co.uk/wiki/Allergic_muscles

Allergy

Allergy is the great mimic. In some ways the immune system is not very clever. It can react to things in only one way – that is, with inflammation. Inflammation causes redness, swelling, pain, heat and loss of function. When you look at a diseased area, you can see those signs, but it does not tell you what is the cause of those signs. So for example, looking at an area of inflamed skin you may not be able to tell if it has been infected, sun-burnt or frozen, had acid spilled on it, or is responding allergically, or whatever. Again, seeing a person with hay fever you may not be able to distinguish this from a head cold. Hay fever sufferers may get a fever too.

You can be allergic to anything under the sun, including the sun. For practical purposes, allergies are split up into allergies to foods, chemicals (including drugs) and inhalants (pollens and microorganisms bacteria, mites, etc).

People with undiagnosed food allergy often initially present with symptoms due to inflammation in the gut (irritable bowel syndrome) and inflammation in the brain (mood swings, depression or brain fog in adults, or hyperactivity in children). However, the inflammation can occur anywhere in the body, resulting in asthma, rhinitis, eczema, arthritis and muscle pain, cystitis or vaginitis, or a combination of symptoms. If the cause is not identified, the inflammation often becomes more generalised. resulting in chronic fatigue.

http://drmyhill.co.uk/wiki/Allergy_to_Foods,_Inhalants_&_Chemicals

Antioxidants

What allows us to live and our bodies to function are billions of chemical reactions in the body which occur every second. These are essential for the production of energy, which drives all the processes of life such as nervous function, movement, heart function, digestion and so on. If all these enzyme reactions invariably occurred perfectly, there would be no need for an antioxidant system. However, even our own enzyme systems make mistakes and the process of producing energy in mitochondria is highly active. When mistakes occur, free radicals are produced. Essentially, a free radical is a molecule with an unpaired electron; it is highly reactive, and to stabilise its own structure it will literally stick on to anything. That 'anything' could be a cell membrane, a protein, a fat, a piece of DNA, or whatever. In sticking on to something, it denatures that something so that it has to be replaced. This means having free radicals is extremely damaging to the body and therefore the body has evolved a system to mop up these free radicals before they have a chance to do such damage and this is called our antioxidant system.

There are many substances in the body which act as antioxidants, but the three most important frontline antioxidants are:

- **coenzyme Q10 (co-Q10):** This is the most important antioxidant inside mitochondria and also a vital molecule in oxidative phosphorylation.

Co-Q10 deficiency may also cause oxidative phosphorylation to go slow because it is the most important receiver and donor of electrons in oxidative phosphorylation. People with low levels of co-Q10 have low levels of energy.

- **superoxide dismutase (SODase)** is the most important superoxide scavenger in muscles (zinc and copper SODase inside cells, manganese SODase inside mitochondria, and zinc and copper extracellular SODase outside cells).
- **glutathione peroxidase:** This enzyme is dependent on selenium and glutathione, a three-amino acid polypeptide, and a vital free radical scavenger in the blood stream.

These molecules are present in parts of a million and are in the frontline process of absorbing free radicals. When they absorb an electron from a free radical, both the free radical and the antioxidant are effectively neutralised, but the antioxidants re-activate themselves by passing that electron back to second-line antioxidants such as vitamins A and beta-carotene, some of the B vitamins, vitamin D, vitamin E, vitamin K and probably many others. These are present in parts per thousand. Again, these are neutralised by accepting an electron, but that is then passed back to the ultimate repository of electrons, namely vitamin C. This is present in higher concentrations.

http://drmyhill.co.uk/wiki/Antioxidants

Arrhythmias

See Dysrhythmias, page 198.

Arthritis

'Arthritis' simply means inflammation in the joints and this results in pain. It names a symptom and is not a diagnosis; it therefore begs the question: what is causing it? Although arthritis has been classified into two types, inflammatory and degenerative, most sufferers usually have a bit of both.

Autoimmunity

Autoimmunity occurs when the immune system has made a mistake. The immune system has a difficult job to do, because it has to distinguish between molecules which are dangerous to the body and molecules which are safe. Sometimes it gets its wires crossed and starts making antibodies against molecules which are 'safe'. For some people this results in allergies, which is a useless inflammation against 'safe' foreign molecules. For others this results in autoimmunity, which is a useless inflammation against the body's own molecules. These are acquired problems – we know that because they become much more common with age. It is likely we are seeing more autoimmunity because of Western lifestyles, diets and pollution.

Chemicals, especially heavy metals, get stuck onto cells and change their 'appearance' to the immune system and thereby switch on inappropriate reactions.
http://drmyhill.co.uk/wiki/Autoimmune_diseases

Brain fog

What I mean by brain fog is:

- Poor short-term memory
- Difficulty learning new things
- Poor mental stamina and concentration – there may be difficulty reading a book or following a film story or following a line of argument
- Difficulty finding the right word
- Thinking one word, but saying another

What allows the brain to work quickly and efficiently is its energy supply. If this is impaired in any way, then the brain will go slow. Initially, the symptoms would be of foggy brain, but if symptoms progress, we end up with dementia. We all see this in our everyday life, with the effect of alcohol being the best example. Short-term exposure gives us a deliciously foggy brain – we stop caring, we stop worrying, it alleviates anxiety. However, it also removes our drive to do things, our ability to remember; it impairs judgement and our ability to think clearly. Medium-term exposure results in moodswings and anxiety (only alleviated by more alcohol). Longer-term use could result in severe depression and then dementia – examples include Korsakoff's psychosis and Wernike's encephalopathy. (Incidentally, these two examples also illustrate how most drug side effects result from nutritional deficiencies – look them up on Wikipedia!)

The cellular form of energy, ATP, along with DNA, is an ancient molecule. It multitasks. It also functions as a neurotransmitter – to be precise a co-transmitter. Other neurotransmitters will not work unless they are accompanied by a molecule of ATP. Improve ATP and you improve all aspects of brain function. Improving ATP delivery is the best treatment for low mood and depression.

http://www.drmyhill.co.uk/wiki/Brain_fog

Candida

See Yeast problems, page 230.

Cell-free DNA

Cell-free DNA is a measure of cell damage. All DNA should be bound up within a nuclear membrane within a cell. DNA in the blood stream, which is not so wrapped up, indicates a cell has burst open as a result of tissue damage.

Chelation therapy

'Chelation' comes from the Greek meaning a 'claw'. Chelation therapy describes any agent which will grab a metal, typically a toxic metal, so it can be excreted in the urine or faeces. A widely used safe chelating agent is DMSA.

Chemical poisoning

The diagnosis of chemical poisoning is suspected from a history of exposures resulting in typical clinical syndromes and confirmed by the appropriate medical tests. There is a series of criteria to be fulfilled to make a confident clinical diagnosis of poisoning by chemicals. The criteria are:

1. The subject was fit and well prior to chemical exposures.
2. There is evidence of exposure to the putative chemicals and toxins.
3. The subject initially developed local symptoms which became worse with repeated exposures.
4. With repeated exposures a typical clinical picture emerges characterised by chronic fatigue syndrome, immune disruption (allergies, autoimmunity, susceptibility to infections), accelerated ageing (so the sufferer gets diseases before their time), neuro-degeneration, diabetes and cancer.
5. Similar patterns of disease are seen in other people working under similar conditions.
6. There is similar factual evidence from other subjects who have been poisoned, such as the Gulf War veterans, sheep-dip poisoned farmers, aerotoxic pilots.
7. There is laboratory evidence of poisoning and effects of that poisoning.
8. There are no other possible explanations for this pattern of symptoms.
9. There is a response to treatment with clinical improvements as a result of detoxification, nutritional and immune support.

http://drmyhill.co.uk/wiki/Chemical_poisoning_-_general_principles_of _diagnosis_and_treatment

Coenzyme Q10

See Antioxidants, page 193.

Detoxification

As part of normal metabolism, the body produces toxins which have to be eliminated, otherwise they poison the system. Therefore, the body has evolved a mechanism for getting rid of these toxins and the methods that it uses are as follows:

- Antioxidant system – for mopping up free radicals. See Antioxidants, page 193.
- The liver – detoxification by oxidation and conjugation (amino-acids, sulphur-compounds, glucuronide, glutathione, etc) for excretion in urine.
- Fat-soluble toxins can be excreted in the bile. The problem here is that many of these are recycled because they are reabsorbed in the gut.
- Sweating – many toxins and heavy metals can be lost through the skin.
- Dumping chemicals in hair, nails and skin, which is then shed.

This system has worked perfectly well for thousands of years. Problems now arise because of toxins which we are absorbing from the outside world. This is inevitable since we live in equilibrium with the outside world. The problem is that these toxins (such as alcohol) may overwhelm the system for detoxification, or they may be impossible to break down (e.g. silicone and organochlorines), or they may get stuck in fatty organs and cell membranes and so not be accessible to the liver for detoxification (for example, many volatile organic compounds). We all carry these toxins as a result of living in our polluted world.

http://drmyhill.co.uk/wiki/Detoxification
http://drmyhill.co.uk/wiki/Detoxing

Diabetes type III

Excessive consumption of sugar, together with insulin resistance, is driving our current epidemics of dementias, and the mechanism of such is closely allied to the mechanisms of damage in type II diabetes. Hence Alzheimer's disease is being called 'diabetes type III'.

DMSA

This is the chelating agent 2-3-dimercapto-succinic acid magnesium salt, used for heavy metal detox. It binds with metals in the body and takes them with it when excreted.

http://drmyhill.co.uk/wiki/Heavy_metal_poisoning

DNA adducts

This test identifies chemicals that have stuck onto DNA. Of course, nothing should be stuck onto DNA – it should be pristine. Anything stuck onto DNA is potentially dangerous. I use this test regularly for patients who have either been exposed to chemicals or developed cancer. However, this test should be employed routinely as a cancer prevention tool. Acumen Laboratories often find toxic chemicals, including lindane, nickel, hair dyes, PBBs (used as fire retardants) and other heavy metals. It is possible to get rid of these toxins, either by using high doses of the beneficial minerals, or using chelation therapy, or doing sweating detox regimes, or a combination of these factors.

http://drmyhill.co.uk/wiki/DNA_adducts

Dysrhythmias

A normal person's heart should beat somewhere between 65 and 80 beats per minute, with the rate slightly speeding up as one breathes in and slightly slowing down as one breathes out. Fit athletes have a slower pulse because, as a result of training, the heart beats more powerfully at rest. A regular beat is achieved by the pacemaker, which is comprised of cells at the top of the heart – that is, within the atria. Our natural, in-built pacemaker generates an electrical pulse, which firstly flows down the top of the heart thereby making the atria contract; there is a small delay whilst the electrical wave flows into the bottom half of the heart, which makes the two ventricles contract. It is this alternate contraction of the atria which fires blood into the ventricles to fill them up, followed by a contraction of the ventricle, which fires blood out of the heart and sends it on its way round the body. One can, therefore, get irregular heart rate or lack of coordination between the atria and the ventricles, or lack of coordination of the ventricles, as a result of disturbances of the pacemaker or the tissues that conduct the wave of electricity away from the pacemaker to the rest of the heart.

Disturbances of the pacemaker and conducting tissue cause a whole variety of heart dysrhythmias, from the heart going too slow or going too fast, to missed beats, irregular beats, or a complete disassociation of heart activity such as atrial fibrillation or even ventricular tachycardias or fibrillations. However, whatever the nature of the disturbance, the fundamental causes are pretty much the same. Many of these disturbances, such as ventricular ectopics, are fairly harmless and do not cause too much trouble. However, you should see them as a warning sign to change your lifestyle and address the underlying factors that are causing them in order that they do not progress to anything more serious.

Electrical disturbances of the heart are caused by: poor blood supply; micronutrient deficiencies; poor energy supply at the cellular level; thyroid disease; and toxic stress. All these need to be investigated and addressed. My general guidance for good health, as outlined throughout this book, may be sufficient. Should you have established dysrhythmias requiring prescription medication, then no changes should be made to medication without informed discussion with your GP and ideally your cardiologist. All dysrhythmias need medical input from your GP or cardiologist but the interventions on my website may be additionally helpful.

http://drmyhill.co.uk/wiki/Heart_Dysrhythmias,_Irregular_Pulse,
 _Missed_beats_and_Palpitations

Energy expenditure

We all have a pot of energy which is available to us to spend over the day. What prevents us spending too much is the symptom of fatigue. We have to spend that pot of energy just to stay alive in 'house keeping' duties, as well as mentally, physically, emotionally or immunologically. If either the pot of energy is too small (because of poor mitochondrial function, poor fuel supply, poor adrenal function, poor thyroid function and so on) or we spend energy wastefully, we can develop chronic fatigue. Of course, the business of pacing is all about spending mental and physical energy judiciously. Many have experienced how energy sapping it is to expend emotional energy. However, I suspect a greatly overlooked cause of wasting of energy is immunological.

http://www.drmyhill.co.uk/wiki/Energy_Expenditure_in_ME
 /CFS:_Immune_wastage_of_energy_and_Rituximab

Enzyme-potentiated desensitisation (EPD)

Enzyme-potentiated desensitisation (EPD) is a vaccine which can be used to desensitise patients to foods, inhalants and chemicals. It has some bacterial antigens. The vaccine has been developed and refined by Dr Len McEwen over the past 30 years. It is supplied to the doctor who mixes the appropriate dose in a sterile environment, immediately prior to dosing. EPD works by manipulating the normal immune processes for creating and turning off allergies.

http://drmyhill.co.uk/wiki/Enzyme_Potentiated_Desensitisation_(EPD)

Epigenetics

Epigenetics is the study of external or environmental factors that turn genes on and off in biological systems. **Methylation** (the addition of a methyl group to a substrate) is catalysed by enzymes and such methylation can be involved in the modification of heavy metals, the regulation of **gene expression**, the regulation of protein function, and RNA processing.

Exercise

Humans, along with all other mammals, evolved living physically active lives. This usually meant long hours of sustained activity, but there would be occasions when maximal energy output was needed, for example, to fight an enemy or bring down prey. It could be argued that most internal metabolism is geared towards physical activity and without this we cannot be fully well.

We need exercise as we need food and water: in just the right amount. Too much risks injury and muscle damage; too little and we degenerate. To maintain optimal fitness, we need steady sustained exercise combined with outbursts of extreme energy. Just as with food, the type of exercise and the amount are critical. After research and practical application, Dr Doug McGuff and John Little produced their book *Body by Science: a research based program for strength training, body building, and complete fitness in 12 minutes a week*. Thanks to their work, we can now see how to exercise most efficiently. We do not want to do so much that we wear out our body (this is what happens with so many athletes – most runners are carrying injuries), but when we do exercise it must be effective to improve cardiovascular fitness. What is so interesting about Little and McGuff's approach is how well this correlates with what we already know about mitochondria, blood sugar control and fats. This approach makes perfect evolutionary sense. I do not see badgers and foxes trotting round my hill every morning to get fit!

Most of the time wild animals are in hiding or feeding quietly. Once a week there will be a predator–prey interaction – the predator must run for his life to get his breakfast, the prey must run for his life! In doing so, both parties will achieve maximal lactic acid burn. This is all that is required to get fit and stay fit.

http://www.drmyhill.co.uk/wiki/Exercise_-_the_right_sort

Far-infrared sauna

Time-honoured methods of detoxification include saunas, Turkish baths and spa therapies, and I recommend all these treatments to my patients. However, the problem with these treatments is that not only do they warm up the skin and subcutaneous tissues, but the whole body is warmed up. This means that chemicals are mobilised from the fat (which largely speaking lies underneath the skin), and when they get into the bloodstream they can cause acute poisoning.

Many of my patients are therefore unable to tolerate these sweating therapies. Furthermore, many sick CFS patients cannot tolerate heat because this increases demands on the heart. In severe CFS, energy delivery to the heart is impaired so it cannot increase its output to cope with the demands of heat.

This is why I became particularly interested in a new technique described in Dr Sherry Rogers' book *Detoxify or Die* (available from Amazon). She advocates a technique called 'far-infrared saunas'. Far-infrared rays constitute the main energy source that comes from the sun and are responsible for warming our skin when we sit in direct sunshine. The rays penetrate several centimetres through the skin and heat up subcutaneous tissues. With enough sun on the skin, the skin will sweat; chemicals from subcutaneous tissues will be mobilised and pass out through sweat. The sunshine does this without heating up the core temperature (although if you lie in the sun for long enough, then your core temperature will eventually rise), therefore chemicals can be mobilised and excreted without causing systemic poisoning. Dr Rogers describes many case histories in her book of patients who, for example, have severe heart disease who would certainly not tolerate a sauna, but who can tolerate FIRS very comfortably.

http://drmyhill.co.uk/wiki/Detoxing

Fermenting gut

The human gut is almost unique amongst mammals: the upper gut is a near-sterile, digesting, carnivorous gut (like a dog's or cat's) to deal with meat and fat, whilst the lower gut (large bowel or colon) is full of bacteria and is a fermenting, vegetarian gut (like a horse's or cow's) to digest vegetables and fibre. From an evolutionary perspective this has been a highly successful strategy – it allows Eskimos to live on fat and protein and other people to survive on pure vegan diets.

Problems arose when humans learned to cook and to farm. This allowed them to access new foods – namely, pulses, grains and root vegetables. These need cooking to be digestible. From an evolutionary perspective this has been highly successful and allowed the population of humans to increase at a great rate. However, carbohydrates have the potential to be fermented in the upper gut with problems arising as detailed below. It is possible that some psychiatric conditions are caused by gut microbes fermenting neurotransmitters to create amphetamine- and LSD-like substances – not my idea but from a Japanese researcher called Nishihara (see References, page 231).

The stomach, duodenum and small intestine should be almost free from micro-organisms (bacteria, yeasts and parasites – that is, 'microbes'). This is normally achieved by: eating a Paleo-ketogenic diet; having an acidic stomach which digests protein efficiently and kills the acid sensitive microbes; then an alkali duodenum, which kills the alkali-sensitive microbes with bicarbonate; then bile salts (which are also toxic to microbes) and pancreatic enzymes to further digest protein, fats and carbohydrates. The small intestine does more digesting and also absorbs the amino acids, fatty acids, glycerol and simple sugars that result.

Anaerobic bacteria, largely bacteroides, flourish in the large bowel, where foods that cannot be digested upstream are then fermented to produce many substances highly beneficial to the body. Bacteroides ferment soluble fibre to produce short-chain fatty acids – over 500 kcals of energy a day can be generated. This also creates heat to help keep us warm. The human body is made up of 10 trillion cells, yet in our gut we have 100 trillion microbes or more – that is, 10 times as many. Bacteria make up 60 per cent of dry stool weight. There are over 500 different species, but 99 per cent of microbes are from 30 to 40 species.

In some people there are bacteria, yeasts and possibly other parasites existing in the upper gut, which means that foods are fermented there instead of being digested. When foods get fermented this can cause symptoms and problems for many reasons such as:

- wind, bloating, heartburn and other digestive problems (so-called irritable bowel syndrome)
- malabsorption
- production of toxins through fermentation or enhanced absorption of toxic metals
- allergy to microbes in the gut (inflammatory bowel disease)
- allergy to microbes at distal sites – arthritis, interstitial cystitis, asthma, urticaria, PMR and many others
- in the longer term – cancer, diverticulitis

http://drmyhill.co.uk/wiki/Fermentation_in_the_gut_and_CFS

Glucagon

Glucagon is the hormone that raises blood sugar levels. It does so by mobilising sugar from the liver (gluconeogenesis) and from fat stores in the body. It does the opposite to insulin. I suspect it is responsible for the symptoms of headache and nausea which often occur when people suddenly swap to low-carbohydrate, high-fat diets and the ratio between glucagon and insulin suddenly changes.

Gout

Gout is one of those conditions that never really made sense to me until I learned that uric acid is an important antioxidant in the bloodstream. What this means is that if levels of other antioxidants fall low, then the body compensates for this by pushing out more uric acid. That is absolutely fine, but the trouble is that if the level of uric acid gets too high, then, being rather insoluble, it precipitates out as crystals in the joint to cause an acute attack of gout. This is very tiresome because acute gout is extremely painful! The immune system does not like these gritty crystals in the joints and produces lots of inflammation to get rid of it and it is this that causes the heat, pain, swelling, redness and loss of function. The diagnosis is made by the characteristic clinical picture of acute, severe joint pain, but one can also get a low-grade generalised arthritis from gout. Blood tests will show high serum uric acid and it is this that gives the game away. Acute attacks are often precipitated by dehydration so uric acid is relatively concentrated.

Any such tendency is made worse where there is a metabolic acidosis (see Acid-alkali balance, page 189), which is an almost inevitable result of Western diets and lifestyles. Acidosis can be calculated from the anion gap.

This gives us a three-pronged approach:

1. Improve antioxidant status in the blood – this is the best approach to treatment (see Antioxidants, page 193).
2. Correct the acidosis.
3. Rehydrate.

http://drmyhill.co.uk/wiki/Gout

Gulf War syndrome (GWS)

GWS is the archetypal environmental illness suffered by any person involved in the Gulf Wars. It was caused by a combination of factors, including:

- Immune insult caused by many different vaccinations (up to 14 in some soldiers) given on the same day
- Chemical warfare – organophosphate chemical weapons were used in the Gulf, notably sarin
- Biological warfare – infectious agents were sprayed onto the troops; the organism was *Mycoplasma incognito*
- Pyridostigmine – this is the 'antidote' to organophosphate poisoning but is toxic in its own right

- Organophosphate pesticides – used for control of sand flies and other insects, were weekly sprayed onto tents
- Fumes from oil-well fires
- Uniforms dipped in organophosphates
- Depleted uranium resulting in radioactive exposures
- Water from drinking and showering often stored in tanks usually used for oil and diesel

This was the most environmentally polluting war in history. Veterans tell me that the chemical alarms were constantly going off but the usual response was to switch the alarm off! Many of the soldiers who came back from the Gulf War with GWS are suffering, amongst other things, from a chronic infection caused by *Mycoplasma incognito*. This was developed as part of germ warfare and it may be that many thousands of the veterans are infected. Treatment is with high-dose doxycycline 200 milligrams daily for six weeks, with further cycles given subsequently. To find out more about mycoplasmal infections and how to test for them, visit the website of the Institute for Molecular Medicine (www.immed.org).

The symptoms of GWS are identical to those of CFS. Recently the Ministry of Defence has admitted that GWS can be caused by organophosphate poisoning. This is not at all surprising to me because the clinical features of GWS are identical to those in my 'sheep dip 'flu' farmers. By taking a careful history I often find evidence of pesticide exposure in CFS patients also – often they had not connected the chemical exposure to their symptoms. Examples include woodworm timber treatments, house fumigation, excessive use of fly sprays/Vaponas and pet flea-treatments.

http://drmyhill.co.uk/wiki/Gulf_War_Syndrome

Hyperventilation

Before I read Stalmatski's book *Freedom from Asthma* I had never understood why humans evolved such an inefficient system of breathing. We inhale most of our recently exhaled air, which to me seemed a nonsense: it is much more efficient to have a one-way flow of air over a surface, like fish do with water over gills. However, there is a good reason. Life evolved over millions of years in an atmosphere rich in carbon dioxide, the waste gas of respiration. Carbon dioxide became essential for normal cell metabolism because cells used carbon dioxide to maintain their optimal pH (acidity). When levels of carbon dioxide in the atmosphere fell, cells had to develop a mechanism for artificially bathing themselves in the right level of carbon dioxide for their efficient metabolism.

And so lungs evolved. Lungs are necessary to keep carbon dioxide levels high in inhaled air and therefore in the blood. The blood is very efficient at gathering oxygen and all arterial blood is 100 per cent saturated with oxygen. But here comes the crunch – oxygen is only readily released from red blood cells to supply oxygen to the tissues in the presence of high levels of carbon dioxide. So what does this mean in practice?

Many patients, particularly asthma patients, but also CFS patients, have a sensation that they are not getting enough oxygen to their tissues. Their response to this is to breathe more deeply. However, blood cannot become more than 100 per cent saturated with oxygen. All that happens is that more carbon dioxide is washed out of the blood. This makes oxygen cling more fiercely to haemoglobin in red blood cells and therefore oxygen delivery to the tissues is made worse. Paradoxically, to improve oxygen supply to the tissues in the short term, you have to breathe less! Breathing less increases carbon dioxide levels and improves oxygen delivery.

Lowering carbon dioxide levels in the blood has other dire effects. It upsets the acidity of the blood and causes what is known in medical jargon as a respiratory alkalosis (but it is driven by acidosis). This causes all sorts of awful symptoms, such as panic attacks, pain, fatigue, feeling spaced out and dizzy, brain fag, brain fog and so on. Again, taking the evolutionary approach, humans used to live a far more active existence. Because we are now so sedentary, we do not need the oxygen supply our lungs have evolved to deliver. We do not produce enough of the waste gas carbon dioxide either. The system is underused and so there is an in-built tendency to breathe too much. This is worsened by stimulants such as excitement (sitting in front of an exciting film, but not using any oxygen up), caffeine, computer games and so on. Hyperventilation is probably extremely common because Western lifestyles tend to result in an acidosis.

http://drmyhill.co.uk/wiki/Hyperventilation

Hypochlorhydria

Hypochlorhydria arises when the stomach becomes leaky and so cannot retain hydrochloric acid – it leaks out as fast as it is pumped in. Alternatively, the stomach becomes less efficient at producing hydrochloric acid. It is a greatly overlooked cause of problems. The stomach requires an acid environment for several reasons:

- Acid is required for the digestion of protein.
- Acid is required for the stomach to empty correctly, and failure to do so results in gastro-oesophageal reflux disease (see page 157).

- Acid is required to sterilise the stomach and kill microbes that may be ingested.
- An acid environment is required for the absorption of certain micronutrients, in particular divalent and trivalent cations such as calcium, magnesium, zinc, copper, iron, selenium, boron and so on.

As we age, our ability to produce stomach acid declines, but some people are simply not very good at producing stomach acid, sometimes because of pathology in the stomach (such as an allergic gastritis secondary to food intolerance), but sometimes for reasons unknown. The stomach is lined with cells that are proton pumps – that is to say they pump hydrogen ions from the blood stream into the lumen of the stomach. Stomach acid is simply concentrated hydrogen ions.

There is a natural tendency for these hydrogen ions to diffuse back from where they came but this is prevented by very tight junctions between stomach wall cells. However, if the gut becomes inflamed for whatever reason, a 'leaky gut' (see page 210) develops and hydrogen ions leak back out. A common cause of inflammation and leaky gut is allergy.

Short-term treatment includes taking: acid supplements, such as cider vinegar; high-dose ascorbic acid with meals; or betaine hydrochloride capsules. Often in the longer term, with the correct diet (low glycaemic index, low allergy potential, smaller meals), getting rid of *Helicobacter pylori* and correcting gut flora, this cures the chronic gastritis and the stomach is again able to produce acid normally.

It is important to mitigate this extra acid with alkali. I suggest using magnesium carbonate 1 gram taken 90 minutes after food, or 1–3 grams last thing at night.

http://drmyhill.co.uk/wiki/Hypochlorhydria

Hypoglycaemia

'Hypoglycaemia' is the term used for blood sugar being at too low a level. To explain how this happens it is necessary to describe how sugar levels are controlled.

It is critically important for the body to maintain blood sugar levels within a narrow range. If the blood sugar level falls too low, energy supply to all tissues, particularly the brain, is impaired. However, if blood sugar levels rise too high, then this is very damaging to arteries and the long-term effect of arterial disease is heart disease and strokes. This is caused by sugar sticking to proteins and fats to make AGEs (advanced glycation end products) which accelerate the ageing process.

Normally, the liver controls blood sugar levels. It can convert glycogen stores inside the liver to release sugar into the blood stream minute by minute in a carefully regulated way to cope with body demands, which may fluctuate from minute to minute. Excess sugar flooding into the system after a meal can be mopped up by muscles, but only so long as there is space there to act as a sponge. This occurs when we exercise. This system of control works perfectly well until we upset it by eating a high-carb diet or not exercising. Eating excessive sugar at one meal, or excessive refined carbohydrate, which is rapidly digested into sugar, can suddenly overwhelm the muscle and the liver's normal control of blood sugar levels.

We evolved over millions of years eating a diet that was very low in sugar and had no refined carbohydrate. Control of blood sugar therefore largely occurred as a result of eating this Paleo-ketogenic diet and the fact that we were exercising vigorously, so any excessive sugar in the blood was quickly burned off. Nowadays the situation is different: we eat large amounts of sugar and refined carbohydrate and do not exercise sufficiently to burn off this excess sugar. The body therefore has to cope with this excessive sugar load by other mechanisms.

When food is digested, the sugars and other digestive products go straight from the gut in the portal veins to the liver, where they should all be mopped up by the liver and processed accordingly. If excessive sugar or refined carbohydrate overwhelms the liver, the sugar spills over into the systemic circulation. If not absorbed by muscle glycogen stores, high blood sugar results, which is extremely damaging to arteries. If we were exercising hard, this would be quickly burned off. However, if we are not, then other mechanisms of control are brought into play. The key player here is insulin, a hormone secreted by the pancreas. This is very good at bringing blood sugar levels down and it does so by shunting the sugar into fat. Indeed, this includes the 'bad' cholesterol LDL. There is then a rebound effect and blood sugars may well go too low – in other words, hypoglycaemia occurs. Low blood sugar is also dangerous to the body because the energy supplied to all tissues is impaired.

Subconsciously, people quickly work out that eating more sugar alleviates these symptoms, but of course they invariably overdo things; the blood sugar level then goes high and they end up on a roller-coaster ride of blood sugar level going up and down throughout the day.

Ultimately, this leads to 'metabolic syndrome' or 'syndrome X' – a major cause of disability and death in Western societies, since it is the forerunner of diabetes, obesity, cardiovascular disease, degenerative conditions and cancer. http://drmyhill.co.uk/wiki/Hypoglycaemia

Hypothyroidism

Underactive thyroid is a very common cause of fatigue, often as a knock-on effect of a general suppression of the hypothalamic-pituitary-adrenal axis – that is, the coordinated functioning of those three glands. Symptoms of hypothyroidism arise for four reasons – the gland itself fails (primary thyroid failure), or the pituitary gland which drives the thyroid gland into action under-functions, or there is failure to convert inactive thyroxine (T4) to its active form (T3), or there is thyroid-hormone receptor resistance. The symptoms of these four problems are the same, but blood tests show different patterns:

- In primary thyroid failure, blood tests show high levels of thyroid stimulating hormone (TSH) and low levels of T4 and T3.
- In pituitary failure, blood tests show low levels of TSH, T4 and T3.
- If there is a conversion problem, TSH and T4 may be normal, but T3 is low.
- In thyroid hormone receptor resistance, there is a high TSH, high T4 and high T3.

There is another problem too, which is that the so-called 'normal range' of T4 is probably set too low. I know this because many patients with low-normal T4 often improve substantially when they are started on thyroid supplements to bring levels up to the top end of the normal range.

http://drmyhill.co.uk/wiki/Hypothyroidism

Inflammation

Inflammation is an essential part of our survival package. From an evolutionary perspective, the biggest killer of *Homo sapiens* (apart from *Homo sapiens*) has been infection, with cholera claiming a third of all deaths, ever. The body has to be alert to the possibility of any infection, to all of which it responds with inflammation. However, inflammation is metabolically expensive and inherently destructive. It has to be, in order to kill infections by bacteria, viruses, parasites or whatever. For example, part of the immune defence involves a 'scorched earth' policy – tissue immediately around an area of infection is destroyed so there is nothing for the invader to parasitise. The mechanism by which the immune system kills these infections is by firing free radicals at them. However, if it fires too many free radicals, then this 'friendly fire' will damage the body itself. Therefore, for inflammation to be effective it must be switched on, targeted, localised and then switched off. This entails extremely complex immune responses; clearly, there is great potential for things to go wrong.

Inflammation is also involved in the healing process. Where there is damage by trauma, there will be dead cells. Inflammation is necessary to clear away these dead cells and lay down new tissues. Inflammation is characterised by heat and redness (heat alone is antiseptic), combined with swelling, pain and loss of function, which immobilises the area being attacked by the immune system. This is necessary because physical movement will tend to massage the infection to other sites.

If one looks at life from the point of view of the immune system, it has a very difficult balancing act to manage. Too little reaction and we die from infection; too much reaction is metabolically expensive and damaging. If switched on inappropriately, the immune system has the power to kill us within seconds, an example of this being anaphylaxis.

http://drmyhill.co.uk/wiki/Inflammation

Kefir

Kefir is a fermented drink made with kefir 'grains' (a yeast/bacterial fermentation starter) and has its origins in the north Caucasus mountains around 3000 BC. It is a useful probiotic because it is rich in *Lactobacillus*, which keeps the lower gut slightly acidic, displaces unfriendly bacteria, is directly toxic to yeast and is anti-inflammatory to the gut. Production of traditional kefir requires a starter community of kefir grains, which are added to the liquid one wishes to ferment. Kefir grains cannot be produced from scratch, but the grains grow during fermentation, and additional grains are produced. Kefir grains can be bought from or donated by other growers. The joy of using kefir is that one sachet can last a lifetime. Furthermore, the best results for probiotics come from using live cultures. I have been growing kefir and it grows well at room temperature. Because dairy products are not evolutionarily correct foods, kefir should be grown on non-dairy foods such as soya milk, rice milk or coconut milk, and who knows what else! Start off with one litre of soya milk in a jug, add the kefir sachet and within about 12–24 hours it should have semi-solid, junket-like consistency. Do not expect it to look like commercial yoghurt, which has often been thickened artificially. Then keep the culture in the fridge, where it ferments further. This slower fermentation seems to improve the texture and flavour. However, it can be used at once as a substitute in any situation where you would otherwise use cream or custard. I often add a lump of creamed coconut which further feeds the kefir, imparts a delicious coconut flavour and thickens the culture. Once the jug is nearly empty, add another litre of soya milk, stir it in, keep it at room temperature and away you go again. I don't even bother to wash up the jug – the slightly hard yellow bits on the edge I just stir in to restart the brew. This way a sachet of kefir lasts for life. One idea I am playing with is the possibility of adding vitamins and minerals to the culture. The idea here is that they may be incorporated into the bacteria and thereby enhance the absorption of micronutrients. You could try this if you do not tolerate supplements well.

http://drmyhill.co.uk/wiki/Kefir

Leaky gut

Leaky gut means that substances which should be held in the gut leak out through the gut wall – this causes many problems:

- Hydrogen ions (i.e. acid) cannot be concentrated in the stomach, leading to hypochlorhydria (see page 205). This causes malabsorption of minerals and vitamin B12. Hypochlorhydria is a major risk factor for fermenting gut since acid helps to sterilise the upper gut. It also is an essential part of protein digestion.
- Allergy – Normally one expects foods to be completely broken down into amino acids (from protein), essential fatty acids and glycerol (from fats) and single sugars or 'monosaccharides' (from carbohydrates). The undigested foods stay in the gut and the small digested molecules pass through the gut wall into the portal blood stream and on to the liver where they are dealt with. However, leaky gut means food particles get absorbed before they have been properly digested. This means large food molecules get into the blood stream. These large molecules are 'interesting' to the immune system, which may mistake them for viruses or bacteria. In this event, it may attack these harmless molecules, either with antibodies or directly with immune cells. This causes inflammation. Inflammation in the gut causes diseases of the gut. Inflammation elsewhere can cause almost any symptom you care to mention. It may switch on allergy or autoimmunity – that is, it is potentially a disease-amplifying process.
- Another problem with small digested molecules or polypeptides getting into the bloodstream is that these molecules may be biologically active. Some of them act as hormone mimics, which can affect levels of glucose in the blood or blood pressure. This is akin to throwing a handful of sand into a finely tuned machine – it makes a real mess of homeostatic (balancing) mechanisms of controlling body activities.

http://drmyhill.co.uk/wiki/Leaky_gut_syndrome

Leiden factor V

This is a genetically inherited disorder that causes an increase in blood clotting. It is the most common hereditary hypercoagulability (prone to clotting) condition amongst European Caucasians.

Lipids, fats and essential fatty acids

The vast majority of cell metabolism takes place on, in or around cell membranes. The structure of cell membranes is identical throughout the animal kingdom. They are made up of fatty molecules which have a water-loving end and a fat-loving end; these combine in a sandwich so the fat-loving end forms the core of the membrane and the water-loving end the outside of the membrane. The structure of the membrane and how liquid it is depends on the fats that are in it. If the composition of membranes changes, then they will either become more stiff or more liquid.

There are a great many effects which result from this, for example increased irritability and sensitivity, which of course could explain many CFS symptoms, such as intolerance of chemicals and foods, intolerance of heat, light and touch, low pain threshold, cardiac dysarrhythmias and so on. Indeed, a great many drugs work because of their effects on changing membrane structure, such as general anaesthetics, tranquillisers, pain killers and anti-inflammatory drugs.

Mitochondrial membranes are different from cell membranes because they have to be a little stiffer in order to hold still the bundles of enzymes called cristae on which oxidative phosphorylation (see page 34) takes place. They have an additional fat – namely cardiolipin – to create this extra stiffness.

Having the correct oils in the diet is essential for energy supply to the brain. Poor energy supply means foggy brain.

http://drmyhill.co.uk/wiki/Lipids,_fats_and_essential_fatty_acids

Magnesium

Magnesium is an essential mineral required for at least 300 different enzyme systems in the body. It is centrally involved in the energy delivery systems of the body, i.e. mitochondria.

Red blood cell levels of magnesium are almost invariably low in patients with CFS. Furthermore, very many patients with CFS benefit from magnesium by injection.

I believe that a low red cell magnesium is a symptom of mitochondrial failure. It is the job of mitochondria to produce ATP for cell metabolism and about 40 per cent of all mitochondrial output goes into maintaining calcium/magnesium and sodium/potassium ion pumps. I suspect that when mitochondria fail, these pumps malfunction and therefore calcium leaks into cells and magnesium leaks out. This, of course, compounds the underlying mitochondrial failure because calcium is toxic to mitochondria and magnesium is necessary for normal mitochondrial function. This is just one of the many vicious cycles we see in patients with fatigue syndromes. The reason for giving magnesium by injection is to reduce the work of the calcium/magnesium ion pump by reducing the concentration gradient across cell membranes.

http://www.drmyhill.co.uk/wiki/Magnesium

Maintaining and restoring good health

I describe my general approach throughout the book, but in summary it consists of the Basic Package viz:

A. Paleo-ketogenic diet
B. Multivitamins, minerals, essential fatty acids
C. Sleep
D. Exercise
E. Sunshine and light
F. Reduce the chemical burden
G. Sufficient physical and mental security to satisfy our universal need to love and care, and be loved and cared for
H. Avoid infections and treat any that arise aggressively

http://drmyhill.co.uk/wiki/The_general_approach_to_maintaining
    _and_restoring_good_health

Malabsorption

The job of the gut is to absorb the goodness from food. To do this, it first has to reduce food particles to a size which allows the digestive enzymes to get at them; then it has to provide the correct acidity then alkalinity for enzymes to work, produce the necessary enzymes and emulsifying agent (bile salts), and move the food along the gut. Finally, the large bowel allows growth of bacteria for a final digestive/fermentative process and water extraction. The gut has a particularly difficult job because it has to identify foods that are safe from potentially dangerous microbes (most are not dangerous but positively beneficial). This explains why 90 per cent of the immune system is gut associated. The innoculation of the gut with these gut-friendly microbes takes place in the first few minutes following birth.

Anything which goes wrong with any of these processes can cause malabsorption. Malabsorption means that the body does not get the raw materials for normal everyday work and repair. Consequently, there is the potential for much to go wrong.

http://drmyhill.co.uk/wiki/Malabsorption

Mercury poisoning

The early symptoms of mercury poisoning can be variable but may include loss of short-term memory, a metallic taste in the mouth (this is difficult since taste is relative and dental amalgam is constantly present) and fine tremor. Mercury may also cause personality changes (like the Mad Hatter from *Alice in Wonderland*, which was written at a time when hatters used mercury in hat-making). It is also toxic to the nerves of the heart and may be a cause of electrical dysrhythmias (palpitations).

Dental amalgam is the commonest source of mercury poisoning. Professor Fritz Lorscheider's work over many years has looked at how mercury leaches out from dental amalgam. At room temperature, mercury is a liquid and in dental amalgam it is not chemically bound into the amalgam, but there as a liquid, albeit a very tough and stiff liquid. He took sheep, filled their molars with dental amalgam which was radioactively labelled and four months later scanned the sheep to see if the mercury had migrated; he discovered that it had deposited in their heart, bones, kidneys and brain. He then looked at what mercury does in the brain. He found that, at concentrations lower than those present in the saliva of a person with amalgam fillings, nerve fibres collapsed because they could not build their essential structure. (For more detail see the link below.)

The pathology he found is similar to Alzheimer's disease, in which neuro-fibrillary tangles are formed. Essentially, Lorscheider's findings tell us that mercury causes Alzheimer's disease. Alzheimer's is also associated with aluminium poisoning and, indeed, aluminium is a very similar metal to mercury in the periodic table of elements. The main source of aluminium is from ant-acids, antiperspirants and cooking foil, pots and pans.

In California, Sweden, Germany and Norway mercury amalgam has been banned.

http://drmyhill.co.uk/wiki/Mercury_-_Toxicity_of_Dental_Amalgam
    _-_Why_you_should_have_your_dental_amalgams_removed

Metabolic syndrome

This is the clinical picture that results from Western diets and lifestyles. The major causes are high-carbohydrate diets and lack of exercise. It is worsened by micronutrient deficiencies, toxic stress and the upper fermenting gut.

The early symptoms include a need to eat regularly (hypoglycaemia), a tendency to go for addictions (sugar, caffeine, nicotine and alcohol), disturbed sleep, mood swings and fatigue.

Metabolic syndrome usually progresses to obesity, hypertension and diabetes. It is the major cause of arterial disease, heart disease, cancer and dementia.

Micronutrients

Micronutrients are substances required in trace amounts for the normal growth and development of living organisms. While these should all be adequately supplied by our diet the problem is that modern Western diets do not deliver. As such, I recommend that everyone take a Basic Package of supplements, which includes a multivitamin supplement, multiminerals, essential fatty acids (omega-6 and -3 in the proportion of 4:1, such as one tablespoon of hemp oil) with additional vitamins D, B12 and C.

A good multivitamin is easy to purchase. However, I have been unable to find a good multimineral preparation which contains all essential minerals in adequate amounts, in the correct proportion and in a form which is is soluble and easily absorbed. So I formulated my own product which has in addition extra vitamin B12 and vitamin D. This physiological Multi Mineral Mix (MMM) is not to be confused with 'Miracle Mineral Solution' (MMS), about which the Food Standards Agency has issued an urgent warning. My MMM is a mix of minerals which you make up in water, and which are all essential for human metabolism. The amounts given below are elemental weights of the pure mineral. These amounts are those considered desirable from modern nutrition research and are mostly above the 'recommended daily amount' (RDA). These RDA amounts were set down in 1941 and are now outdated. If better preparations become available or I learn more about essential minerals, then the composition of MMM may change. The newest formulation contains B12 1 milligram per gram (mg/g) of MMM and vitamin D, 1,000 IU (international units) per gram.

- Calcium (as calcium chloride) – 60 mg
- Magnesium (as magnesium chloride) – 70 mg
- Potassium (as potassium chloride) – 40 mg
- Zinc (as zinc chloride) – 6 mg
- Iron (as ferric ammonium chloride) – 3 mg
- Boron (as sodium borate) – 2 mg
- Iodine (as potassium iodate) – 0.3 mg
- Copper (as copper sulphate) – 0.2 mg

- Manganese (as manganese chloride) – 0.2 mg
- Molybdenum (as sodium molybdate) – 40 mcg
- Selenium (as sodium selenate) – 40 mcg
- Chromium (as chromium chloride) – 40 mcg
- Vitamin B12 – 1,000 mcg/g
- Vitamin D (as cholecalciferol) – 1,000 IU

Dosage: the daily dose of MMM is one gram (one blue scoop) per two stone (12.5 kilograms) of body weight to a maximum of 5 grams (five scoops) per day. This dose assumes that you get nothing from food. However, as your diet improves and deficiencies are corrected the dose can be reduced – most people need just 2–3 grams daily for maintenance of good health.

The daily dose should be dissolved in cold water – half a pint of water per 1 gram of the mix (the maximum dose made up in three pints of water) and taken throughout the day. You should start off with just half a pint of mix daily and build up slowly to allow your stomach to adjust to the changes; otherwise it may cause nausea and loose bowel movements. Ideally, use with ascorbic acid (vitamin C) to optimise absorption. The juice of half a lemon makes this more palatable. It also makes one drink water; this is something many people forget to do. MMM is suitable for all age groups, including babies and pregnant women. The dose is not critical as there is a wide margin of safety for all essential minerals. The mix is 100 per cent active ingredient with no additives, colourings, flavourings or bulking substances. The formula is completely stable and will last for many years. Keep the lid tightly screwed on to the jar; otherwise moisture from the air may be absorbed and the minerals change colour. This does not matter, but the contents may go hard or discolour slightly.

Vitamin C can be taken with the MMMs or at night. The idea here is that vitamin C helps to keep microbes in the upper gut at a low level (you can never completely sterilise the upper gut). Vitamin C kills all microbes, including viruses.

http://drmyhill.co.uk/wiki/Nutritional_Supplements

Minerals

You could argue that we all die ultimately from mineral and vitamin deficiencies. People who traditionally live to a great age are often found living in areas watered by streams from glaciers. Glaciers are lakes of ice which have spent the previous few thousand years crunching up rocks. Therefore the waters coming from the glaciers are rich in minerals. This is used not just to drink but to irrigate crops and to bathe in. These people therefore have had excellent levels of micronutrients throughout life. Given the right raw materials, things do not go wrong in the body and ageing is slowed. For example:

- Low magnesium and selenium is a risk factor for heart disease
- Low selenium increases risk of cancer
- Copper is necessary to make elastic tissue – deficiency causes weaknesses in arteries leading to aneurysms
- Low chromium increases the risk of diabetes
- Good antioxidant status (vitamins A, C, E and selenium) slows the ageing process
- Superoxide dismutase enzymes require zinc, copper and manganese to function
- Iodine is necessary to make thyroid hormones and is highly protective against breast disease
- The immune system needs a huge range of minerals to work well, especially zinc, selenium and magnesium
- Boron is highly protective against arthritis
- Magnesium is required in at least 300 enzyme systems
- Zinc is needed for normal brain development; a deficiency at a critical stage of development causes dyslexia
- Any deficiency of selenium, zinc, copper or magnesium can cause infertility
- Iron prevents anaemia
- Molybdenum is necessary to detox sulphites

The secret of success is to copy Nature. Civilisation and Western diets have brought great advantages, but at the same time have been responsible for escalating death rates from cancer, heart disease and dementia. I want the best of both worlds. I like my warm kitchen, fridge, wood-burning cooker, computer and telly, but I want to eat and live in the environment in which primitive man thrived.

http://drmyhill.co.uk/wiki/Minerals

Multiple chemical sensitivity

Multiple chemical sensitivity (MCS) is an inevitable part of modern Western lifestyles because we are inevitably exposed to toxic chemicals and Western lifestyles are pro-inflammatory. Chemicals have huge potential to do harm, and if the body senses this it will set up an early warning system. It achieves this by giving you unpleasant symptoms when you are exposed to such a chemical. In low doses, chemicals can be detoxified in the body and do not cause problems. If our defences are overwhelmed, the chemical will cause a poisoning. The body recognises this and remembers the chemical, so in the future, when there are tiny, non-poisonous exposures, the alarm bells ring with symptoms. This is fine if it is just one or two chemicals causing minor symptoms – for example, if I smell perfume I will sneeze, but with larger doses I suffer a foggy brain. The mechanism of this is the same as the mechanism for viral infection and subsequent immunity.

Problems arise when there is sensitivity to many chemicals and the warning symptoms are severe. Some people can have anaphylactic reactions to chemicals, with complete collapse. For some it involves a sudden and major flare of their fatigue, muscle symptoms, migraine or whatever. What this means in practice is that chemical sensitivity and toxicity go together. People with chemical sensitivity have been 'poisoned' somewhere in the past and are likely to have an ongoing toxic load. This is why detox regimes are part of the treatment I advocate for CFS.

http://drmyhill.co.uk/wiki/Multiple_Chemical_Sensitivity_(MCS)
    _-_Principles_of_Treatment

Muscle stiffness

Muscle stiffness is a symptom seen when muscles cannot move quickly without accompanying pain or spasm. Sufferers have to move slowly. They soon work out that after the muscle has not been used for some time – for example, on rising from sleep, or from having sat in one position for some time – their first movement has to be particularly slow, gentle and tentative. Moving too quickly brings about acute pain and possibly spasm.

Thanks to the work of Dr McLaren-Howard, we know the possible mechanisms for this stiffness include:

1. For muscles to relax they require magnesium and for muscles to contract they require calcium. Any imbalance of this – that is, too much calcium or too little magnesium – very much increases the tendency to spasm and contraction.
2. Modern diets are low in magnesium and high in calcium and this will increase the tendency to spasm.
3. Other dietary indiscretions will also raise intercellular calcium levels. Calcium is held inside cells via a binding protein and this is stimulated by cyclic AMP and insulin. The two dietary problems which induce

these enzymes are caffeine and carbohydrates respectively. Therefore, a Western diet will tend to predispose towards muscle stiffness.

4. Rheumatic patches may well present with the symptom of stiff muscles.
5. We have the issue of allergic muscles (see page 192).
6. Once a person has developed a tendency to muscle spasm and pain, we then get a learned response. The brain anticipates that the muscle will go into spasm if moved too quickly and therefore all movements are generally slowed down to prevent this from happening. It may well be that therapies known to be effective for stiff muscles, such as Pilates, Bowen technique, massage and other such manipulations, are re-educating the brain into realising that it is now 'safe' to move freely. However, they will be much more effective if the underlying physical causes are also addressed.
7. There is clearly a neuro-psychological element. The brain is also responsible for muscle tone and neurological problems such as Parkinson's disease will result in muscle stiffness or even spasticity. Psychological stress will also tend to increase muscle tension and worsen an underlying tendency. Diazepam is one of the most useful muscle relaxants.
8. Exercise – the right type may well be a factor.

http://drmyhill.co.uk/wiki/Muscle_Stiffness

NAD – nicotinamide adenine dinucleotide

Nicotinamide is vitamin B3, vital to make NAD which is an essential part of energy delivery mechanisms within mitochondria. Though present in meat, eggs and whole grains, it is such a common deficiency that we should all be taking a supplement (at least 500 mg daily, possibly 1500 mg slow release) to slow the ageing process.

Naltrexone

The idea behind using low-dose naltrexone is to stimulate the production of endogenous (the body's own) opiates. These have disease-modifying effects in a wide range of conditions and there is now good evidence for this.

Naltrexone on its own has very little effect on the body. Typically, it is used to reverse the effects of poisoning by opiates such as morphine, and is the perfect antidote to, for example, morphine or a morphine-like substance which may be used for darting and tranquillising wild animals. They will wake up within a few minutes if injected with naltrexone. The usual dose of naltrexone to treat opiate poisoning is 50 milligrams. The daily dose of naltrexone for our purposes is 1–4 milligrams.

Naltrexone is available in the UK on prescription, either from your GP or from a private practitioner. It comes in several forms – as capsule, liquid or transdermal cream.

http://drmyhill.co.uk/wiki/Low_dose_naltrexone

Neutralisation

Neutralisation is a technique to turn off allergies. A small amount of antigen (food, inhalant or chemical) is injected into the skin to elicit a skin reaction and possibly symptoms. The injection is repeated at progressively greater dilutions until the 'neutralising' dose is found, at which level there is no skin reaction and symptoms are switched off. The patient then self-treats daily with this neutralising dose, possibly with drops under the tongue or injections. It is a laborious technique since every antigen has to be neutralised individually – furthermore the neutralisation end points can change. However, it is helpful to identify allergies where there is uncertainty.

Nickel

Nickel (Ni) is a nasty toxic metal and a known carcinogen. It is one of the metals we see most commonly in toxicity tests – it appears stuck onto DNA, stuck on to translocator protein and is often present in blood at high levels. Nickel is a problem because biochemically it 'looks' like zinc. Zinc deficiency is very common in people eating Western diets, so if the body needs zinc and it is not there, it will use look-alike nickel instead. But nickel does not do the job and, indeed, gets in the way of normal biochemistry. Zinc is an essential co-factor in many enzyme systems from alcohol dehydrogenase to zinc carboxypeptidase, so there is enormous potential for harm from nickel. Nickel sensitivity is very common and often diagnosed from rashes from jewellery, zips, watches etc. What we know from people with chemical sensitivity is that they often have toxic loads of those things they are sensitive to. So nickel sensitivity often equates with nickel toxicity.

Nickel is unavoidable if you live a Western lifestyle. Many industrial processes release nickel into the atmosphere.

- Stainless steel contains 14 per cent nickel; this includes cookware and eating utensils. Use cast-iron pans, glass or ceramic.
- Jewellery – used because it is such a versatile, malleable metal. Well absorbed with piercing.

- Catalytic converters in cars release fine particulate nickel into the atmosphere – so fine that it cannot be filtered out by the lining of the bronchus, so it is well absorbed by inhalation and easily gets into blood vessels. Here it triggers inflammation and arterial disease.
- Cigarette smoke.
- Medical prostheses.

http://drmyhill.co.uk/wiki/Nickel_-_a_nasty_toxic_metal

NO/ON/OO cycle – pronounced No Oh No!

This is a self-perpetuating pro-inflammatory cycle described by Professor Martin Pall. It is a central part of all processes involving inflammation. I think of it as a fire which is driven by many possible factors, including poor micronutrient and antioxidant status, toxic stress and immune activation (infections, autoimmunity and allergy). It perpetuates many vicious cycles – for example, poor mitochondrial function results in excessive free radicals being produced which, if not mopped up by antioxidants, further damage and inhibit mitochondrial function.

The No-Oh-No cycle (appropriately named!) seems to have a momentum of its own, and once fired up it needs all possible interventions to damp the blaze down.

Nutritional supplements

See Micronutrients, page 214.

Organophosphate (OP) poisoning

This is a remarkably common but under-diagnosed problem because we are all constantly exposed to organophosphates, including glyphosate – this (Round-up is the best known product) is generally regarded as safe, but this is not so.

Different people have different symptoms of OP poisoning. Symptoms depend partly on how much OP they have been exposed to, whether they have had single massive exposure, or chronic sub-lethal exposure, whether it has been combined with other chemicals and, how good their body is at coping with toxic chemicals. Symptoms divide into the following categories:

No obvious symptoms at all – A government-sponsored study at the Institute of Occupational Medicine that looked at farmers who regularly handled OPs but who were complaining of no symptoms, showed that they suffered from mild brain damage. Their ability to think clearly and problem solve was impaired.

Sheep dip 'flu (mild acute poisoning) – This is a 'flu-like illness which follows exposure to OPs. Sometimes the farmer just has a bit of a headache, feels unusually tired or finds he can't think clearly. This may just last a few hours to a few days and the sufferer recovers completely. Most sufferers do not realise that they have been poisoned and put any symptoms down to a hard day's work. It can occur after dipping, but some farmers will get symptoms after the slightest exposure, such as visiting markets and inhaling OP fumes from fleeces.

Acute organophosphate poisoning – This is the syndrome recognised by doctors and Poisons Units. Symptoms occur within 24 hours of exposure and include collapse, breathing problems, sweating, diarrhoea, vomiting, excessive salivation, heart dysrhythmias, extreme anxiety, etc. Treatment is with atropine. You have to have a large dose of OP to have this effect (such as, drink some of the dip!) and so this syndrome is rarely seen.

Intermediate syndrome – This occurs 1–3 weeks after exposure and is characterised by weakness of shoulder, neck and upper leg muscles. It is rarely diagnosed because it goes unrecognised.

Long-term chronic effects – These symptoms develop in some susceptible individuals. They can either occur following a single massive exposure, or after several years of regular sub-lethal exposure to OPs. Essentially there is an acceleration of the normal ageing process with arterial disease, heart disease, cancer and dementia presenting at a young age.

The treatment follows the same principles as for any chemical poisoning (see Chemical poisoning, page 196).

Fortunately, most farmers are intelligent and realise the above state of affairs, but the lack of street credibility and help from government agencies makes this illness a social and financial disaster area.

http://drmyhill.co.uk/wiki/Organophosphate_Poisoning

Osteoporosis

Osteoporosis is a modern disease of Western society. Primitive societies eating Paleo-ketogenic diets do not suffer from osteoporosis. So the underlying principle for avoiding osteoporosis is that we should mimic primitive cultures eating a Paleo-ketogenic diet and living a toxin-free life. This does not mean you need to run around half naked in a rabbit-skin loin cloth depriving yourself of the pleasures of twenty-first-century Western life. We need to cherry pick from the good things of all civilisations.

To make good quality bone you need the raw materials (Paleo-ketogenic diet and supplements), the ability to absorb minerals (an acid stomach), the drive to lay these down in bone (exercise, vitamin D, DHEA) and an alkali body to prevent minerals being washed out in urine (magnesium carbonate at night). I have collected 'before and after' bone density scans of 14 patients doing these regimes. In all cases, the bone density has remained the same or increased. So whilst the numbers are small the statistics are powerful.

Dairy products and calcium supplements alone make osteoporosis worse. This is because calcium in isolation blocks the absorption of other essential minerals, such as magnesium. Vitamin D is the key to calcium – it promotes the absorption of calcium (and magnesium) and ensures its deposition in bone.

The medical profession would have us believe that the only important constituent of bone is calcium. Actually bone is made up of many different minerals, including magnesium, calcium, potassium, boron, silicon, manganese, iron, zinc, copper, chromium, strontium and maybe others. For its formation bone also requires a whole range of vitamins, essential fatty acids and amino acids.

http://www.drmyhill.co.uk/wiki/Osteoporosis

Pain

Although pain seems like 'a pain', actually it is essential for our survival. Pain protects us from ourselves. It prevents us from damaging our bodies. Indeed, people who are born with no pain perception look as if they have been traumatised – they are covered in cuts, bruises and sores, because they are unaware that they are damaging themselves. Pain is the local method of avoiding damage – it makes us protect the affected part of the body and makes us keep it still so that healing and repair can take place. If pain becomes more generalised then pain is accompanied by fatigue. What this means is that chronic pain and chronic fatigue go hand in hand and therefore so should treatment. We learn through experience what is painful; this makes us avoid those painful experiences and therefore protects our bodies.

Although it is desirable to learn about pain, this can also cause problems because if the underlying causes of the pain are not identified we 'learn' more pain. In the ideal situation, we damage our bodies with say a cut or bruise and the local pain makes us care for that damaged area by protecting it and keeping it still so that healing and repair can take place. With healing the pain goes. If the root source of the pain is not identified, it creates a problem because then the pain increases. The body naturally thinks that increasing pain means we will take more care, identify the source of the pain, keep the limb more still and therefore the body winds up the pain signal to try to elicit the appropriate response. Effectively we learn to feel more pain because there is an upgrading of this pain response. This is not a psychological effect – this actually occurs within the cells themselves. This makes it very important to identify causes of pain early on in any disease process and allow time for healing and repair, otherwise the pain will get worse.

http://drmyhill.co.uk/wiki/Pain

Paleo-ketogenic diet

Human beings evolved over millions of years eating particular foods. Neanderthal man was a carnivore and only ever ate meat, fish and shell fish. Fat would have been a treasured food. The carbohydrate content would have been, for much of the year, zero. More recently Paleolithic man expanded the diet to include root vegetables, fruits, nuts and seeds which he could scavenge from the wild, but even these would only be available occasionally in season. It is only in the last few thousand years since the Persians, Egyptians and Romans that we began farming, and grains and dairy products were introduced into the human diet. A few thousand years from an evolutionary point of view is almost negligible. Many people have simply failed to adapt to cope with carbohydrates and dairy products and it is very likely that these foods cause a range of health problems in susceptible people.

Modern studies on ancient tribes who continue to eat a Paleo-ketogenic diet show that these people do not suffer from diabetes, obesity, heart disease or cancer. If they can survive the ravages of the cold, infectious diseases, childbirth and war wounds, then these people live healthily to a great age. I am coming to the view that whatever our medical problem may be, or even if we simply want to stay well, we should all move towards eating a Paleo-ketogenic diet based on protein (meat, fish, eggs), fat and vegetable fibre. Recent Western diets get 70 per cent of their calories from wheat, dairy products, sugar and potato and it is no surprise that these are the major causes of modern ill health such as cancer, heart disease, diabetes, obesity and degenerative disorders. Traditional Chinese diets have no dairy products, no gluten grains, no alcohol and no fruit.

http://drmyhill.co.uk/wiki/Stone_Age_Diet

Pancreatic function

The pancreas is a large gland which lies behind the stomach and upper gut. It has two major functions of clinical importance. Firstly, it acts as an endocrine organ to produce insulin and other hormones essential for the control of blood sugar. Secondly, it has an exocrine function to produce enzymes essential for the digestion of food. These enzymes include those to digest proteins, fats and starches and to work best they need an alkali environment. When food is present in the duodenum and jejunum, the gall bladder contracts, sending a bolus of bile salts which combines with bicarbonate and pancreatic enzymes to allow digestion to take place in the duodenum and jejunum.

If the pancreas does not produce sufficient digestive enzymes and bicarbonate, then foods will not be digested. This can lead to problems downstream. Firstly, foods may be fermented instead of being digested and this can produce the symptom of bloating due to wind, together with metabolites such as various alcohols, hydrogen sulphide and other toxic compounds. Secondly, foods are not fully broken down so that they cannot be absorbed and this can result in malabsorption.

Where there is severe pancreatic dysfunction it is obvious because the stools themselves become greasy and fatty, foul smelling, bulky and difficult to flush away. Where there is malabsorption of fat, there will be malabsorption of essential fatty acids such as the omega-3 and omega-6 fatty acids, and there will be malabsorption of fat-soluble vitamins such as vitamins A, D, E and K. If foods are poorly digested, this results in large antigenically interesting molecules appearing downstream, which alerts the immune system and could switch on allergies – that is, poor digestion of food is a risk factor for allergy.

Where there is poor pancreatic function, digestive aids can be very helpful. I use pancreatic enzymes together with magnesium carbonate 90 minutes after food (not with food since we need a 90-minute window of time of acidity for stomach function). High-dose pancreatic enzymes have revolutionised the treatment of cystic fibrosis.

http://drmyhill.co.uk/wiki/Pancreatic_exocrine_function

Prion disorders

I think of prion disorders as protein cancers. Prions are proteins which are normally present in the body and perform essential functions. However, if they come into contact with a particular toxin or heavy metal or another twisted prion (rotten apple effect), then they too twist and distort. When they twist in such a way that they cannot be broken down by the body's enzyme systems, they cause problems because the body has to dump them as it cannot break them down. Pathologically this is known as amyloid. This results in deposition of these indigestible proteins and this can occur anywhere in the body.

Cancers, of course, are simply cells which replicate themselves and build up to cause problems. Viruses are strips of DNA which replicate themselves and build up in the body to cause problems. Difficulties arise when they literally get in the way of the body and stop it functioning normally. Although amyloid can occur anywhere in the body, the biggest problem is in the brain, partly because it is a closed box and therefore there is not any room for all this excess protein to be dumped and partly because each part of the brain is unique and any loss of function is quickly noticed. So these protein cancers tend to cause problems which may take many years to develop and so far the medical profession has no method of slowing down this process. The conditions they cause include Alzheimer's disease, Parkinson's disease, Creutzfeldt-Jacob's disease, motor neurone disease, and multisystem atrophy (MSA). We are currently seeing an epidemic of these conditions – the number of people suffering from it is increasing fast. Not my words but the words of Professor Colin Pritchard, professor of epidemiological medicine at Southampton University. These diseases are an inevitable part of Western lifestyles and diets high in sugar and refined carbohydrate. Indeed, Alzheimer's has been dubbed 'type III diabetes' of the brain.

http://www.drmyhill.co.uk/wiki/Prion_disorders

Probiotics

In a normal situation free from antiseptics, antibiotics, high-carbohydrate diets, bottle feeding, hormones and other such accoutrements of modern Western life, the gut flora is safe. Babies start life in mother's womb with a sterile gut (although interestingly there is some evidence that their gut becomes innoculated before birth through transfer of microbes across the placenta!). During the process of birth, they become inoculated with bacteria from the birth canal and perineum. These bacteria are largely bacteroides which cannot survive for more than a few minutes outside the human gut. This inoculation is enhanced through breast-feeding because the first milk, namely colostrum, is highly desirable substrate for these bacteria to flourish. We now know that this is an essential part of immune programming. Indeed, 90 per cent of the immune system is gut associated. These essential probiotics programme the immune system so that they accept them and learn what is beneficial. A healthy gut flora therefore is highly protective against invasion of the gut by other strains of bacteria or viruses. The problem is that there is no probiotic on the market that supplies bacteroides for the above reasons. If we eat probiotics which have been artificially cultured, for a short while the levels of these probiotics in the gut do increase. However, as soon as we stop eating them, levels taper off and may disappear. Ideally, for bacteria to be accepted into the normal gut and remain, they have to be programmed first through somebody else's gut (in this case, mother's).

So, when it comes to repleting gut flora, there are two ways that we can go about this – either we can take probiotics very regularly (and the cheapest way to do this is to grow your own probiotics) or to take bacteroides directly. Indeed, this latter technique is well established in the treatment of *Clostridium difficile* (a normally fatal gastroenteritis in humans) and interestingly in idiopathic diarrhoea in horses. In the latter case horses are inoculated with the bacteria from the gut of another horse. These ideas have been developed further by Dr Thomas Borody with his ideas on faecal bacteriotherapy, which can provide a permanent cure in cases of ulcerative colitis, severe constipation, *Clostridium difficile* infections and pseudomembranous colitis. The reason this technique works so well is because the most abundant bacteria in the large bowel, bacteroides, cannot survive outside the human gut and cannot be given by any other route.

The gut flora is extremely stable and difficult to change. Therefore if you are going to take probiotics, you have to be prepared to take them for the long term. Many preparations on the market are ineffective. Those found to be most effective are those milk ferments and live yoghurts where the product is freshly made. It is not really surprising. Keeping bacteria alive is difficult and it is not surprising that they do not survive dehydration and storage at room temperature.

So your best chance of eating live viable bacteria is to buy live yoghurts or drinks. These can be easily grown at home, just as one would make home-made yoghurt. If you cannot grow easily from a culture, then it suggests that the culture is not active, so this is a good test of what is and is not viable. I have tried to culture on soya and coconut milks from dried extracts with very poor success rates – suggesting that the dried extracts are not viable in the gut.

The use of probiotics is already established practice in animal welfare and probiotics are actively marketed to the horse industry for this very reason. Furthermore, probiotics are routinely used in the pig industry to prevent post-weaning diarrhoea. Anyone who has to take antibiotics for any reason should take these cultures as a routine to prevent 'super-infection' with undesirable bugs. These cultures are also an essential part of re-colonising the gut following gut eradication therapy.

http://drmyhill.co.uk/wiki/Probiotics

Rebounding

Sitting or lying still allows bone to break down. To stimulate bone formation requires changing forces through bone. This is efficiently achieved with a mini-trampoline – gentle bouncing up and down results in rapidly changing gravitational fields (none at the top of the bounce, much more at the lowest point).

Salt pipes

It was observed that miners working in the salt mines were protected from lung disease, including allergic and infectious conditions. This was in marked contrast to most other miners. The effect is due to salt in inhaled air – perhaps an anti-infection or anti-inflammatory mechanism. Salt pipes should be standard treatment for any respiratory condition.

Sleep

Humans evolved to sleep when it is dark and wake when it is light. Sleep is a form of hibernation when the body shuts down in order to repair damage done through use, to conserve energy and to hide from predators. The normal sleep pattern that evolved in hot climates is to sleep, keep warm and conserve energy during the cold nights and then to sleep again in the afternoons when it is too hot to work and to hide away from the midday sun. As humans migrated away from the Equator, the sleep pattern had to change with the seasons and as the lengths of the days changed.

After the First World War a strain of Spanish 'flu swept through Europe killing 50 million people worldwide. Some people sustained neurological damage and for some this virus wiped out their sleep centre in the brain. This meant they were unable to sleep at all. All these unfortunate people were dead within two weeks and this was the first solid scientific evidence that sleep was as essential for life as food and water. Indeed, all living creatures require a regular 'sleep' (or period of quiescence) during which time healing and repair take place. You must put as much work into your sleep as your diet. Without a good night's sleep on a regular basis all other interventions are undermined.

http://drmyhill.co.uk/wiki/Sleep_is_vital_for_good_health

Superoxide dismutase (SODase)

SODase is one of the most important antioxidant enzymes which mop up free radicals. It is the most important superoxide scavenger in muscles. Deficiency can explain muscle pain and easy fatiguability in some patients. Normal levels of SODase are dependent on good levels of copper, manganese and zinc.

http://www.drmyhill.co.uk/wiki/SODase_(superoxide_dismutase)_studies

Syndrome X

A pre-diabetic state, also known as 'metabolic syndrome', when blood sugar levels see-saw between too high and too low in the presence of excessively high levels of insulin. See Hyoglycaemia, page 206.

Tachydysrhythmias (literally fast, abnormal rhythms)

This term means the heart is beating too fast considering the demands placed on it. For diagnostic purposes it is helpful to feel the pulse to see if the rate is regular or irregular. Fast and regular could be an excess adrenaline effect and may indicate a serious problem. Irregular is always abnormal and needs full medical investigation.

Toxins

These are substances that are dangerous to the body because they inhibit normal metabolism, damage the structure of the body or are wasteful of its resources. Organophosphates, for example, inhibit oxidative phosphorylation. Toxic metals can stick onto DNA and trigger cancer; they also stick onto proteins to trigger prion disorders. Products of the upper fermenting gut require energy and micronutrients for the liver to deal with them. Volatile organic compounds may need methylating to detoxify them and this is a drain on folic acid and vitamin B12.

Toxins come from the outside world (exogenous) and the inside world (endogenous). Exogenous toxins include POPs (persistent organic pollutants), metals, radiation (most of this comes from the medical profession), toxic halides (fluorides, bromides) and many more. A major source of toxic stress is from prescription medication. Endogenous toxins come from the fermenting gut, natural toxins in foods (e.g. lectins, mycotoxins), breakdown products of normal metabolism, from inflammation, and other such.

Modern Western lifestyles mean we are inevitably exposed to chemicals. See my website for a checklist of exogenous toxins and their sources:

http://drmyhill.co.uk/wiki/Chemical_poisons_and_toxins

Transdermal micronutrients

I see many patients for whom we know what the micronutrient deficiency is that causes their problem, but giving those micronutrients by mouth does not help, or indeed makes them worse. What I suspect is getting in the way is the gut. For micronutrients to get into the body to do good they must first get there! To achieve this we need the ability to digest and absorb them and also the energy to do this. I suspect the latter is a problem for many of my severe CFS patients. Food allergy, the upper fermenting gut and poor stomach, liver and pancreatic function may all be problems. This may explain why so many of my sick patients do well on injections of micronutrients.

To get round this problem I use transdermal preparations to be sprayed onto the skin. A key ingredient is DMSO – this passes through skin like a knife through butter and carries through everything dissolved within it. DMSO is a naturally occurring, organic, sulphur-containing molecule, derived from tree bark and closely related to MSM (a useful treatment for arthritis). The early clinical feedback has been encouraging.

Transdermal magnesium seems to be especially effective in muscle, joint, tendon and connective tissue problems. I suspect the mechanism of this is that magnesium reduces the friction within tissues.

http://drmyhill.co.uk/wiki/Transdermal_micronutrients

Translocator protein function

Translocator protein is the little postman who picks up ATP from within mitochondria and delivers it through the mitochondrial membrane to the cell where it is needed for energy. ATP breaks down to ADP releasing energy for the cell to use. Our little postman then picks off the ADP and returns it to the mitochondia back across the mitochondrial membrane. Indeed, mitochondrial membranes are 80 per cent composed of these wonderful little postmen. (Actually, I suspect that they are mainly postwomen as things generally work quite well!)

Vitamin D and sunshine

Western cultures have become almost phobic about any exposure of unprotected skin to sunshine. This phobia is based on the perceived risk of skin cancers. However the two skin cancers which are known to be caused by sunshine, namely basal and squamous cell cancers, are easily diagnosed and treated – people very rarely die from these tumours.

The most serious skin cancer is melanoma. This does not appear most commonly on sun-exposed skin. Schools of thought now believe melanoma is not caused by sunshine. Indeed, sunshine is highly protective against all cancers – the key is to tan but not burn. In efforts to avoid burning, the US Environmental Protection Agency is currently advising that ultraviolet light, and therefore sunlight, is so dangerous that we should 'protect ourselves against ultraviolet light whenever we can see our shadow'. This is a nonsense.

Sun exposure is essential for normal good health in order to produce vitamin D – and partly as a result of current recommendations, we are seeing declining levels of vitamin D. There is an interesting inverse correlation between sunshine exposure, vitamin D levels, and incidence of disease as one moves away from the Equator. Even correcting for other factors, such as diet, there is strong evidence to show that vitamin D protects against osteoarthritis, osteoporosis, bone fractures (vitamin D strengthens the muscles thereby improving balance and movement and preventing falls), cancer, hypertension, hypercholesterolaemia, diabetes, heart disease, multiple sclerosis and vulnerability to infections. Multiple sclerosis is a particularly interesting example of a possible vitamin D deficiency disease. Indeed, mice bred for susceptibility to multiple sclerosis can be completely protected against development of this disease by feeding them high doses of vitamin D.

Human beings evolved over hundreds of thousands of years in equatorial areas and were daily exposed to sunshine. Dark skins evolved to protect against sun damage. However, as hominids migrated north, those races which retained their dark skins were unable to make sufficient vitamin D in the skin and did not survive. Only those hominids with paler skins survived. Thus the further away from the Equator, the paler the skin became. Races in polar areas survived because they were able to get an alternative source of vitamin D from fish and seafood.

http://drmyhill.co.uk/wiki/Vitamin_D_and_Sunshine

Yeast problems and candida

Yeast is one of the common fermenting microbes in the upper gut and is part of the upper fermenting gut issue (see page 201). Yeast problems are an inevitable problem of Western diets, which are high in carbohydrates. The problem is worsened by antibiotics, the Pill and HRT.

Problems may arise initially because yeast numbers build up, sometimes to produce overt infections such as oral thrush, perineal thrush or skin tinea infections (ringworm, athlete's foot, fungal toenails, tinea, etc). With chronic exposures there is the potential to sensitise to yeast and that causes much worse problems, characterised by itching, pain and inflammation. Psoriasis may be allergy to yeast; ditto chronic cystitis and interstitial cystitis.

http://drmyhill.co.uk/wiki/Yeast_problems_and_candida

References

Who am I?

1. Myhill S, Booth NE, McLaren-Howard J. Chronic fatigue syndrome and mitochondrial dysfunction. *International Journal of Clinical and Experimental Medicine* 2009; 2(1): 1–16; Booth NE, Myhill S, McLaren-Howard J. Mitochondrial dysfunction and pathophysiology of myalgic encephalomyelitis/chronic fatigue syndrome (ME/CFS). *International Journal of Clinical and Experimental Medicine* 2012; 5(3): 208–20; Myhill S, Booth NE, McLaren-Howard J. Targeting mitochondrial dysfunction in the treatment of myalgic encephalomyelitis/chronic fatigue syndrome (ME/CFS) – a clinical audit. *International Journal of Clinical and Experimental Medicine* 2013; 6(1): 1–15.

Introduction

2. Choo KY. America's healthcare system is the third leading cause of death. *World Health Education Initiative.* (Last accessed November 17, 2017) http://www.health-care-reform.net/causedeath.htm
3. Siegel-Itzkovich J. Doctors' strike in Israel may be good for health. *British Medical Journal* 2000; 320: 1561. doi:10.1136/bmj.320.7249.1561
4. Newman NM, Ling RS. Acetabular bone destruction related to non-steroidal anti-inflammatory drugs. *Lancet* 6 July 1985; 326(8445): 11–14.

Chapter 1: Symptoms

5. Nishihara K. Disclosure of the major causes of mental illness – mitochondrial deterioration in brain neurons via opportunistic infection. *Journal of Biological Physics and Chemistry* 2012; 12: 11–18. doi:10.4024/38NI11A.jbpc.12.01

Chapter 2: Mechanisms and tests

6. Nishihara K. Disclosure of the major causes of mental illness – mitochondrial deterioration in brain neurons via opportunistic infection. *Journal of Biological Physics and Chemistry* 2012; 12: 11–18. doi:10.4024/38NI11A.jbpc.12.01

7. Rashid T, Ebringer A. Autoimmunity in rheumatic diseases is induced by microbial infections via crossreactivity or molecular mimicry. *Autoimmune Diseases* 2012; 2012: Article ID 539282 doi:10.1155/2012/539282

8. Turkel H, Nusbaum I. *Medical Treatment of Down Syndrome and Genetic Diseases*, 4th ed. Southfield, MI: Ubiotica, 1985.

Chapter 3: The tools of the trade

9. Browne SE. The case for intravenous magnesium treatment of arterial disease in general practice: review of 34 years of experience. *Journal of Nutritional Medicine* 1994; 4(2): 169–77.

10. Hoffer A, Saul AW, Foster HD. *Niacin: the real story: learn about the wonderful healing properties of niacin*. North Bergen, NJ: Basic Health Publications, 2012; Hoffer A, Saul AW. *Orthomolecular Medicine for Everyone: megavitamin therapeutics for families and physicians*. Laguna Beach, CA: Basic Health Publications, 2008.

11. Kaufman W. *The Common Form of Joint Dysfunction*. 1950; Saul AW. Taking the cure: the pioneering work of William Kaufman: Arthritis and ADHD. *Journal of Orthomolecular Medicine* 2003; 18(1): 29–32.

12. Joint Formulary Committee. *British National Formulary* Vol 69. Pharmaceutical Press, 2015.

Chapter 4: Treatment

13. Porta M. Persistent organic pollutants and the burden of diabetes. *Lancet* 12 August 2006; 368(9535): 558–59. doi:10.1016/S0140-6736(06)69174-5

14. Beral V, Million Women Study Collaborators. Breast cancer and hormone-replacement therapy in the Million Women Study. *Lancet* 9 August 2003; 362(9382): 419–27.

15. van Steenis D. Airborne pollutants and acute health effects. *Lancet* 8 April 1995; 345(8954): 923. doi:10.1016/S0140-6736(95)90034-9

16. Rashid T, Ebringer A. Autoimmunity in rheumatic diseases is induced by microbial infections via crossreactivity or molecular mimicry. *Autoimmune Diseases* 2012; 2012: Article ID 539282 doi: 10.1155/2012/539282

17. Hermon-Taylor J. Mycobacterium avium subspecies paratuberculosis, Crohn's disease and the Doomsday scenario. *Gut Pathogens* 14 July 2009; 1(1): 15. doi:10.1186/1757-4749-1-15

18. Syddall HE, Sayer AA, Dennison EM, et al. Cohort Profile. The Hertfordshire Cohort Study: *International Journal of Epidemiology* 1 December 2005; 34(6): 1234–42. doi:10.1093/ije/dyi127

Index

About the Author

Dr Sarah Myhill MB BS, the author, qualified in medicine (with Honours) from Middlesex Hospital Medical School in 1981 and has since focused tirelessly on identifying and treating the underlying causes of health problems, especially the 'diseases of civilisation' with which we are beset in the West. She has worked in the National Health Service and private practice and for 17 years was the Hon. Secretary of the British Society for Ecological Medicine, which focuses on the causes of disease and treating through diet, supplements and avoiding toxic stress. She helps to run, and lectures at, the Society's training courses and also lectures regularly on organophosphate poisoning, the problems of silicone, and chronic fatigue syndrome. Visit her website at www .drmyhill.co.uk